The Raindrop Resource Guide
for Oily Families

I0135612

Christina G. Hagan, M.Ed, LCCI, LMBT

Table of Contents

Dedication

This book is dedicated to all those who like me, want to know more, more, more about essential oils and Raindrop.

Acknowledgments

Thank you Gary Young for having the insight to create this technique!

Thank you Dr. Stewart and Lee for having the dream of bringing this technique into every home and creating the Center for Aromatherapy Research and Education. It is your influence that has opened my eyes to the truth and possibilities about essential oils and the love of our creator.

Thank you to my amazing and ever patient husband, Brian who continually supports my dreams and visions and is always willing to be my demo without complaint.

Thank you to my sweet daughter Joy who can always be counted on for helping in this Raindrop journey when I ask her, for giving the best hugs ever and cheering me on when I need it.

Thank you to my mom and dad for being willing to support me whenever needed, even when not asked.

Thank you to ALL of those who shared your Raindrop insight with me and allowed me to include your nugget of wisdom in this book. I am thrilled that your insight will be shared with other Raindroppers. This will offer great support for those who like you, love this technique and see the value in it.

Photo Credits: Thank you Steve Stryker for your beautiful cover photo! Those photos you took many years ago are my favorite Raindrop photos and I am so thankful that I can use this one on the cover.

About the Author

Christina G. Hagan, LMBT, LCCI, MEd, certified instructor and licensed massage therapist, has been teaching and offering the Raindrop Technique® since 2006.

She is excited to be playing a role in enhancing your Wellness Independence with Adapting Raindrop books and on line programs. Her goal is to support others so that they can be more confident and independent in their use of this flexible and effective wellness tool, Raindrop!

Who is this Resource Guide for?

This Raindrop Resource Guide is written for all the Oily Families who incorporate essential oils into their day to support their total health. This is for those who have learned Raindrop either from Gary Young, at Convention, in a three-day or hour class, from their upline, from a video or book, and used it occasionally with family and friends with the goal of total wellness support.

Thank You for Your Contribution!

I have a lot of information, tips and concepts to share with you about Raindrop, but you know what, I know that I don't know it all! There are others who have had more experience in different wellness arenas than I have had, so I added what they shared with me. When I came across a 'Golden Nugget', comment in Adapting Raindrop Facebook Group, I just had to share it with you too. I am thankful for their permission in allowing me to add their quote and name in this Raindrop Resource Guide.

Do you Love Giving Raindrop?

If you love giving Raindrops and find that you are giving them often to people outside of your immediate family, then you may want to consider becoming a Certified Raindrop Technique Specialist / Licensed Spiritual Healer (CRTS/LSH) or Massage Therapist! Did you know that in most states in the United States, it is illegal for someone to 'rub a body' and charge money for it? Yes, it is! So giving a Raindrop and then charging for that Raindrop when you don't have a 'license to touch' may be illegal in your state or county.

You can learn more about how to become a CRTS/LSH by visiting www.RaindropTraining.com. You are welcome to join me for a CARE Intensive or Raindrop class by visiting my website www.AdaptingRaindrop.com and choosing "Live Classes".

Please Share this Guide with Your Oily Friends

I hope you find The Raindrop Resource Guide for Oily Families so useful that you let your Oily Friends know about it. No part of this Resource Guide may be reproduced, transmitted or copied for public or private use.

This is not Intended to Treat, Diagnose or Prescribe

Part 1

Tailoring the Oils

Chapter One: Time to Answer Those Questions

I put this resource guide together for you, a fellow Raindropper for three reasons:

My initial push to create a resource guide like this stemmed from my experience as an Instructor with C.A.R.E. (The Center for Aromatherapy Research and Education). Every time I taught Raindrop, I was asked great questions from the students. Those questions often have a similar vein, "How do you do Raindrop on someone if…" or "What do you do if you have a client that…"

I gave as many tips as possible, but I never had enough time to answer all those questions. That would easily have taken another few hours, which we didn't have in our 'action-packed' C.A.R.E. Intensives!

Once the class was over and the attendees went home and practiced Raindrop, I would then receive more questions sent by text or email, "I have a client who has…" or "I did a Raindrop and my client…"

I've saved many of those questions and hope to offer advice or direction in this book to give Raindroppers the background and confidence to answer many of these questions on their own.

The second reason I put this resource guide together is because I simply LOVE Raindrop and see this as a fluid technique that can be used in a WIDE variety of ways. We are so accustomed to seeing and learning the Basic Raindrop (which I refer to as 'The Basic Recipe'), and many people stop there. I'd like to offer you concepts of how this beautiful technique can be adapted to support the wide variety of people who would benefit from the health supporting quality essential oils offer when delivered in this method.

The third reason for this *Raindrop Resource Guide* is when Gary Young taught Raindrop to an audience of thousands, when Raindrop is demonstrated at convention, when uplines teach it to their downline or when learning from a DVD, there is little or no chance to ask questions.

Raindrop is simply a method of applying oils on the feet and spine. It is a versatile tool that can be used to support the total health of your friends and family. People who attend these events and classes have questions that come up when they start applying this technique at home, and they don't have a place to go to ask for help. I hope this guide will not only answer those questions for you, but will also give you fresh ideas on how to change, adapt or tailor Raindrop to fit the specific and ever-changing needs of your friends and family.

How I View Raindrop

If you look at the theory behind Raindrop, you'll see why it is such a versatile and flexible technique.

Looking at the picture on the next page, notice how the nerves exit the spine and travel through the body to innervate or support various organs, systems or muscle groups in your body.

The molecules of essential oils are tiny electrically charged molecules that are transdermal. Transdermal means that these molecules are absorbed into your body very quickly. Once these oil molecules are absorbed, they enter your blood, lymph, cells and nerves.

In Raindrop, the essential oils are applied or dropped on the spine since the spine is where all the nerves originate.

Being that essential oil molecules are electrical in nature, the theory is that they can travel along the nerves and are 'delivered' to the organs, systems and muscles that the nerve innervates.

Very similar to a subway, the nerve carries the essential oil molecule right to the organ that the nerve supports. When you apply oils on the spine, as in Raindrop, we are using this super quick and efficient delivery system.

I use this 'essential oil subway system technique' in many applications, not just when giving a Raindrop. One example is when my digestive system needed support last year. Instead of applying my essential oils to my belly button, tummy or taking oils orally, I applied the oils along my spine. I rubbed the oils along vertebras L2 to S2. That is where the nerves exit the spine and support my digestive system.

I've used this method many times for various reasons, all with good results.

When you are applying oils along your spine, as in Raindrop, you are using the 'essential oil nerve subway system'. This is just another of the many ways you can use your essential oils. Give this technique a try with one or two oils and see how this delivery system works for you. Feel free to share your thoughts and comments in 'Adapting Raindrop' Facebook Group.

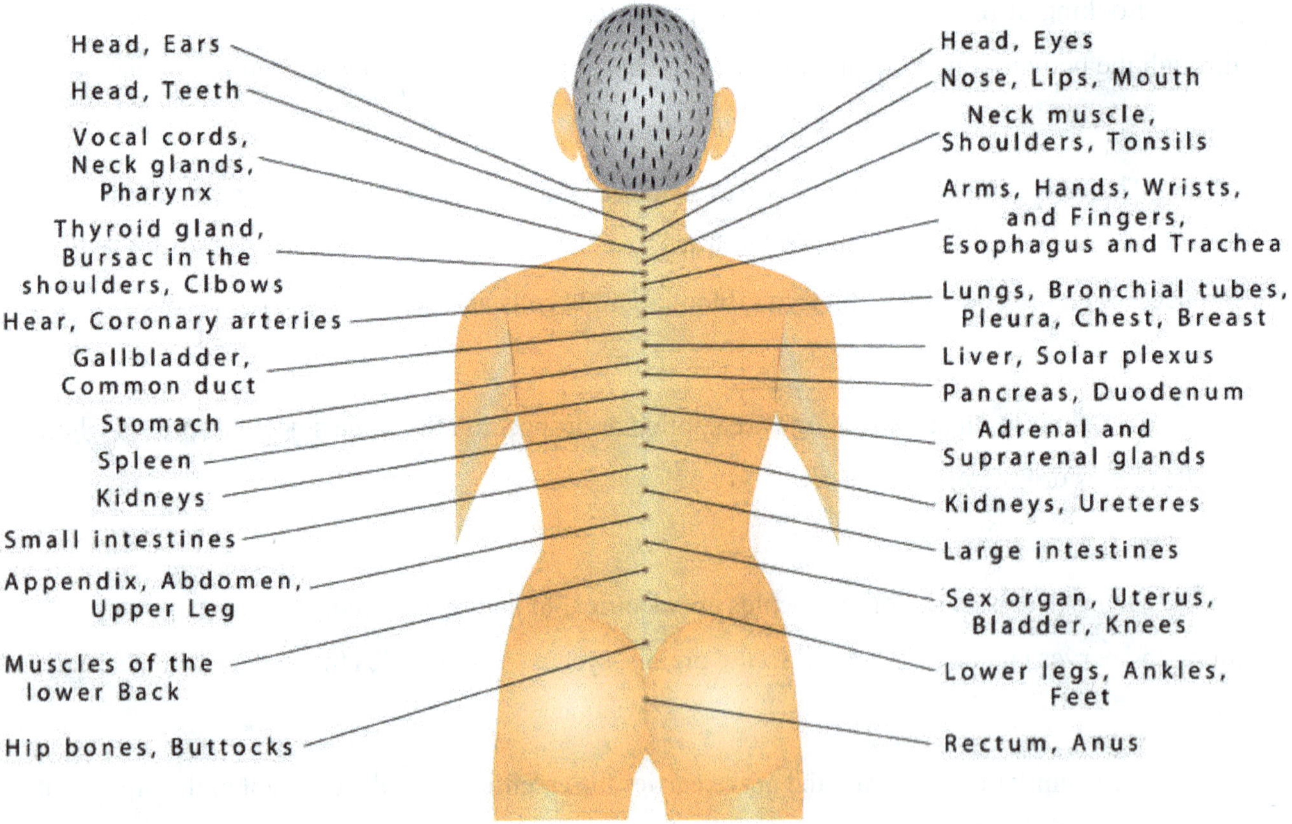
Head, Ears
Head, Teeth
Vocal cords, Neck glands, Pharynx
Thyroid gland, Bursac in the shoulders, Clbows
Hear, Coronary arteries
Gallbladder, Common duct
Stomach
Spleen
Kidneys
Small intestines
Appendix, Abdomen, Upper Leg
Muscles of the lower Back
Hip bones, Buttocks
Head, Eyes
Nose, Lips, Mouth
Neck muscle, Shoulders, Tonsils
Arms, Hands, Wrists, and Fingers, Esophagus and Trachea
Lungs, Bronchial tubes, Pleura, Chest, Breast
Liver, Solar plexus
Pancreas, Duodenum
Adrenal and Suprarenal glands
Kidneys, Ureteres
Large intestines
Sex organ, Uterus, Bladder, Knees
Lower legs, Ankles, Feet
Rectum, Anus

I Wish I Could Ask Gary Young His Thoughts…

Some people I know feel that Raindrop, as designed by Gary Young, is a complete modality and does not need any 'adapting' or changing in any way. From what I understand, as Gary was demonstrating the technique to others at meetings, trainings and conventions, he changed Raindrop to fit the person he was demonstrating on. He often forgot that he was supposed to be in 'teacher mode' during these demonstrations and went into 'healer mode'. This is why Gary would do one set of oils, or different techniques each time he demonstrated Raindrop.

This inconsistency led to some confusion and discourse when people discussed "The best way to do Raindrop is"… or "THIS is THE way Gary taught it!"

In his book *Essential Oils Integrative Medical Guide*, there is a chapter about Raindrop with pictures and directions. Page 228 is often overlooked, but it gives us insight into one of the ways Gary Young was showing us how Raindrop can be adapted. I'll discuss this further in chapter 3.

I'm sorry I missed my opportunity to chat with Gary about how he felt about adapting or changing this effective method of essential oil application, known by millions as The Raindrop Technique®.

Even though I did not have a chance to speak to him face to face, I feel that I received quite a few nudges from him because as this idea for a resource guide and repository was blooming in my head, I could NOT put it aside for the many reasons a busy, self-employed mom would have. I HAD to complete this, NO MATTER WHAT. As the interest in 'Adapting Raindrop' has grown so quickly, I take that as a spiritual thumbs up from Gary. My heart and spirit are beyond excited and jazzed when I think about how many people will benefit from learning these tips and concepts, and I appreciate the gentle nudges!

What We'll Cover Together in This Resource Guide

This resource guide is divided up into three parts:

In Part 1, we'll cover what I call 'The Basic Recipe' for Raindrop and how that recipe can be tailored to fit your Receiver's current needs.

We'll discuss detoxing. One of the beauties of Raindrop Technique is that it is a cleansing and detoxing technique, but that can be its downfall too. Let's detox gently with grace instead of unintentionally and unexpectedly having too strong of a detox.

We'll look at how to add other Essential Oils to Raindrop to support the Receiver either physically or emotionally. You'll learn how to find a substitute oil if you don't have an oil or if your Receiver is allergic to an oil.

Then, as you get more comfortable with the idea of modifying Raindrop, we will look at how to replace some of the essential oils used in the 'Basic Recipe' of Raindrop so you can tailor your Raindrop to fit the current needs of your Receiver. I'll show you my 'System Supporting Raindrop' chart, which will guide you in creating a Raindrop designed to support a specific system.

In Chapter 5, we'll discuss tailoring your base oil choice.

In Part 2, you'll learn about four different options for giving Raindrop if you don't have a massage table. I'll give you some tips on what to do if your Receiver gets stuffy sinuses from lying face down for so long. I'll also address how and why to modify for pregnancy. If you would like, there is a link where you can request to have access to these videos for each option in Part 2. If a picture is worth a thousand words, I thought a video would be at least worth a million! You can request access to them by going to https://adaptingraindrop.com/oilyfamvideos/

Part 3 is all about Special Considerations of your Receivers. This is where I expect this resource guide will grow and develop as more people share with me, through AdaptingRaindrop.com what they have done that has been helpful for their Receivers. I get so excited at the thought that this will be an evolving resource guide for you and me!

The final chapter is all about additional resources and links for you to find Raindrop tools, more education and connections with other Raindroppers and how you can contribute to this growing resource guide.

Okay! Are you ready? Let's start!

Chapter Two: The Basic Recipe

When you are talking Raindrop, there is a basic set or what I call, the 'Basic Recipe' of oils that are used. These were chosen by Gary Young when he developed this oil application technique in the 1980's. His oil choices, of course, are fantastic! They address all the systems of the body and offer a beautiful combination of Phenols, Monoterpenes and Sesquiterpines. These are three molecules found in essential oils that are what help us to receive the support and healing that Raindrop offers.

A quick breakdown of the quality of these molecules are:

Phenols

- Clean off the receptor sites in our cells, dislodging toxins, sugar, and the 'yuck' we are exposed to in our modern world
- Fight invaders (viruses, bacteria, yeast)
- Support our immune system
- Warming to the skin

Monoterpenes

- Bring forth the correct information in our DNA
- Cleansing
- Support healing
- Balancing

Sesquiterpenes

- Remove the incorrect information in our DNA
- Oxygenating
- Mood elevating

If you look at the oils that are used in the Basic Recipe you'll see there are a lot of cleaners used.

Oil	P, M or S
Valor	Monoterpenes & Sesquiterpenes
Oregano	Phenols
Thyme	Phenols
Basil	Phenols
Wintergreen	Phenols
Marjoram	Monoterpenes
Cypress	Monoterpenes & Sesquiterpenes
Peppermint	Phenols

Cleaning is a good thing. We want to cleanse and detox our bodies. The cleansing of our receptor sites on our cells offers the ability of our cells to receive information from messenger caring molecules floating around our bodies. When we have good information between the organs and cells of our bodies, we have health, and that is our goal, right?

What I see is that when people use the Basic Recipe even with the greatest of intentions, they may unknowingly help their Receiver detox too much too fast, which can lead an uncomfortable and unpleasant experience.

Is Our Receiver Ready For A Detox?

When people are detoxing a lot, they often can experience a headache, skin rash, upset tummy or diarrhea. These are known as Herxheimer reactions or a healing crisis.

My personal feeling is detoxing is good, but it is important to know if the Receiver is expecting a detox. Did they come to see you for a detox or just to relax? You need to know what their goals are and are they prepared for the possibility of a detox.

As someone who is offering Raindrop Technique® Massage in my wellness practice, I feel it is of utmost importance that I respect the goals and intention of the Receiver.

I also feel that I need to take into consideration that many people are toxic and don't know it. Just asking someone, "Are you carrying a toxic load?" most likely will not give you the information that you are looking for. I need to ask questions with intention behind it.

As essential oils are becoming more popular and widely used, so is Raindrop (oh yeah!). That means, we need to gain information from the Receiver so we have a greater chance of giving them the outcome that they are expecting.

If you agree with this so far, wonderful, we are literally on the same page!

Once we determine what the goals are of the Receiver, based on their answers, we then may need to adjust the quantity of oils used and we may even change the oils that are used.

As someone who is giving Raindrop to your kids or close family, most likely you have an idea of the answers already. You were probably the one who pulled out the oils and said, "Lay down, I'll give you a Raindrop!"

Even with close family like this, I still want you to consider these questions because thinking about these topics will allow you to make tailored oil choices.

When you are working with downline, friends or people you don't know as well, I want you to ask these questions. Since you are not giving a health history for Receivers to fill out like I do at my office, you can simply have a chat before the Raindrop and ask these questions to your Receiver. It is a nice way to get to know them, know their goals and tailor their Raindrop to fit their current needs.

The Questions To Ask

When I first started doing Raindrop, I did not change the oils or amount used. I stuck with the 'Basic Recipe' because that was what I was taught. Many of the people who I gave Raindrop to enjoyed it, but there were some who detoxed, and detoxed *a lot*. They were not expecting to detox that much, I was surprised too. Even though they enjoyed the experience of receiving a Raindrop, they did not like how they felt after. If I had asked them the questions I am going to share with you in this resource guide, then I would have tailored their Raindrop to fit them for that session. They would have experienced a gentle detox versus an unexpected, unwanted grand detox that kept them at home for a few days.

During the past fourteen years that I've been offering Raindrop and teaching Raindrop, I have noticed an increase in allergies, pharmaceutical use and toxin load. I love how Raindrop supports us in so many ways, but it is because of the increase of ill health that I feel it is important to adapt our Raindrops to fit our Receivers. I want my Receiver to detox slowly and have a pleasant experience so they will return again for more Raindrop sessions to continue their health journey. If they detox too fast like some of my first clients did, without the education or planning for the detox, they could have a negative view of Raindrop and essential oils. Then that would mean that the supportive health benefits of the oils may be lost to them.

This is what prompted me to start changing the amount of oil used. We know that 'more is not always better' and that' less is more' when it comes to essential oil use, so why can't we take that same idea to Raindrop?

I started asking questions too. I wanted to get to know my Receiver more than my massage Health History revealed and get a better understanding of what their toxic load might be like. I also took this time to explain why I was asking these questions. When I explained that their answers might reveal that they could be holding on to toxins, this made my clients think about their health in a new way too.

In my head, I categorized their answers as colored flags. I'm going to use these flag colors here to help us discuss what considerations we should take for each kind of flag.

We have Red Flags, Yellow Flags and Green Flags answers.

Red Flags let me know that this person is most likely toxic and I need to adjust the amount of Essential Oils used so they don't have more of a detoxing experience than they signed up for.

Yellow Flags tell me that I most likely will need to pull back a bit on the amount of Essential Oils used.

Green Flags give me the idea that I do not have to worry so much about this person overly detoxing. I probably don't have to reduce the amount of essential oil used.

Eight Questions + Eight Flags = A Tailored Raindrop

Now, as a mom who is giving Raindrop to her family, many of these questions you know already. I know you are not going to drill your 5-year-old with these eight questions, but it is the concepts behind the questions that I want you to understand.

First question

"What are the goals in giving this Raindrop today?"

> *"I hear many things. Sometimes it's to rest and restore, sometimes it's to realign, sometimes they say just to be quiet and receive healing, it's all about their intent and that becomes my intent. It's powerful when taken the time to ask we see many more results."*
>
> Sherian McCoy

This first question not only plays a huge role in how we can tailor our Raindrop to that person, but it gives intention for both Receiver and Giver. This question gets the Receiver involved with their Raindrop experience and outcome.

As an Oily Family, perhaps you are not going to ask that question to a young child; most likely as the Giver you know the intention. Even if you don't need to ask this question out loud to your Receiver, think on it. The answer can lead to some fantastic oil choices that can then give you a tailored Raindrop. You'll learn more on this in the following chapters.

Possible Answers
- Immune support
- Relaxation
- Muscle Support
- Respiratory Support

Second Question

"What is your job?" "What do you do during the day?"

As a mom, you are not going to ask this question to your kids or husband, you already know the answer. If this is their first Raindrop, it is important to take this concept into account. Thinking about how many toxins a person is routinely exposed to will give us an idea of the amount of toxins they have in their body to release. Think about your past and current jobs. Did you have a job that exposed you to a lot of toxins, such as a hairdresser? What about your husband?

Jobs that routinely expose someone to a lot of toxins get 'Red' flags in my head. That means we'll be planning on reducing the amount of oils used for this person. Jobs that may or may not expose someone to a lot of toxins get a 'Yellow' Flag. Those whose employment offers little exposure to toxins or their lifestyle is a healthy and organic one, get a 'Green' Flag.

This is a question that can impact teens too. Has this teen been using commercial hair care, nail polish and dying her hair purple and pink? Perhaps this teen is a swimmer and spends every day in a chlorinated pool. Both activities add to their toxic load.

Common Professions and their 'Flags':

(R) - Hairdresser

(R) - Nail tech

(R) - Automotive repair

(Y) - Chiropractor

(Y) - Librarian

(G) - Naturopath

(R) =	Red Flag
(Y) =	Yellow Flag
(G) =	Green Flag

Third Question

"How often do you eat fast food?"

This question also gives us an idea of our Receiver's possible toxic load. When it comes to your family, you already know the answer. Be honest.

If you are doing a Raindrop for a friend of a friend, ask them this question.

Possible Answers:

(R) - For Lunch, I always grab fast food and a soda.

(Y) - Once a week, I'll grab something for dinner with the kids.

(G) - I make all my meals at home only using organic ingredients.

The more fast food someone eats, the more toxic load they will be holding on in their body. So for those who eat out often, I will consider reducing and/or diluting the oils used in Raindrop.

Fourth Question

"How often do you have a bowel movement?"

This is an important question or concept to consider because you need to know how your Receiver's exits are working. When the phenols in the essential oils do their detoxing job and your Receiver's exits are not moving, where are those toxins going to go? If there is a backup in their large intestines, and your Receiver is not having regular bowel movements, then those toxins that are released are going to have to find another exit route. A person with sluggish exits has a greater chance of getting a rash from their detox since that colon is backed up and moving slow.

As a mom, you know that answer for your little ones. But, as your kids get older you may not know, especially when they hit the teen years! How about your hubby? How well do you know his BM patterns? Having an open and honest "poop" discussion not only can help you tailor your

Raindrop, but it can also lead to an important conversation, which may have huge long term health impacts.

Possible Answers:

(R) - Well... I go about once a week.

(Y) - I usually go once a day but lately it has been about a few times a week.

(G) - I go 1 or 2 times a day.

For the Receiver who goes once a week, I am going to reduce and/or dilute the oils used in Raindrop. I can also use this information to tailor my oil choices to support my Receiver's digestive system. I may also choose to delay my Raindrop and instead offer to look through the *Essential Oil Desk Reference* with them. Together we can learn about available supplements meant for colon support. Perhaps together, you decide that working on colon health first is a better choice. Once that exit is working regularly, then they are ready to experience their Raindrop.

Fifth Question

"How much water do you drink a day on average?"

This question goes right with question 4. If your Receiver is not cleansing their body with water, then that lets us know that they are holding on to toxins.

When your kids are little, you most likely know this answer. As your kids grow, you probably will need to ask them. This simple question could also lead to important daily health changes. This is a good question for both parents to consider too in the beginning of your oily journey as you are starting to use more oils and experience Raindrop.

Possible Answers:

(R) - I hate water, I only drink diet soda and energy drinks.

(Y) - I drink about two to three 8 oz bottles a day.

(G) - I drink about six to eight 8 ounce bottles of water a day.

Hydration plays a huge role in how you respond to the oils. When people are not drinking water, or not even drinking liquid throughout the day, they most likely will be on the dehydrated side. Dehydration leads to reduced bowel movements and reduced lymph movement. When bowel movements and lymph are slowed down, this will slow down the elimination of toxins. I would reduce and/or dilute essential oils used in Raindrop for a Receiver who does not drink water throughout their day.

Sixth Question

"Tell me about your essential oil use? How long have you been using them, and how do you use them?"

Moms will know this answer because most likely, it is mom that introduced the oils into the home! Just know that the newer your family or family members are to oils, the more you want to reduce or dilute during your first Raindrop experiences.

Possible Answers:

(R) - I don't use them, you do.

(Y) - We just started using them a month ago. They are diffused daily and I just started putting Thieves on my feet every day to support my immune system. I do love those oils.

(G) - I've been using oils for over 6 years. I diffuse, put on my feet and take them in a capsule now and then in the wintertime.

Seventh Question

"Have you had Raindrop before?"

If someone has not experienced Raindrop before, then you don't know what their response is to the oils.

Usual Answers:

(R) - No

(Y/G) - Yes

I give a mental Red Flag for people who have not experienced Raindrop so that I make sure to reduce and/or dilute for their first Raindrop. Always, no matter how long they have used oils or how much they use their oils. If it is their first Raindrop, I reduce and dilute.

Eighth Question

"Do you have any allergies to citrus, wheat, coconut or nuts?

Usual Answers:

(R) - Yes

(G) - No

If someone does have an allergy to one of the choices given above, then it is time to adjust your oil or base oil choices.

I have a client who is allergic to citrus. That means I can't use Joy® or Peace 'n Calming® on her. To be safe, I stick with the singles with her and do not use blends. When you are at home, you can be more vigilant with allergies and oil choices, or you can just stick to singles like I do.

Valor® has a base oil Caprylic/capric triglyceride. This is basically a safe base oil for topical use. It's usually made from combining coconut oil with glycerin. Only people who are highly allergic to coconut have a problem with this base oil.

OrthoEase® has Fractionated Cocos nucifera (Coconut) oil as the first ingredient. It also contains Triticum vulgare (Wheat) germ oil, Prunus amygdalus dulcis (Sweet almond) oil, Vitis vinifera (Grape) seed oil and Olea europaea (Olive) fruit oil.

Here Is A Quick Review Of The Eight Questions.

1. What are your goals with receiving this Raindrop today?

2. What do you do during the day? What is your job?

3. How often do you eat fast food?

4. How often do you have a bowel movement?

5. How much water do you drink a day on average?

6. Tell me about your essential oil use? How long have you been using them and how do you use them?

7. Have you had a Raindrop before?

8. Do you have any allergies to citrus, wheat, coconut or nuts?

When You Do the Math

Using the 'Raindrop Basic Recipe', let's do the math and see how many drops of essential oil are used.

3 drops per foot x 8 oils = 48 drops

4 drops on the back x 8 oils = 32 drops

For a total of 80 drops of essential oil.

That really is quite a lot of essential oil for someone who is new, or totally new to essential oils.

When someone has a few 'Red Flags', this is when we want to reduce and/or dilute their Raindrop. Let's look at some ways you can reduce and dilute Raindrops for your family and friends.

Reduce and Dilute Tips

How do we adapt the 'The Basic Recipe' to reduce the chances of someone detoxing too much? Here are some ideas. Use your judgment to decide which one you will use. You can always use more than one of these ideas.

- Apply base oil on the spine before you add any essential oils. This slows down the absorption of the oils, especially the first few, which are the 'phenolic' cleansing oils.

- Simply reduce the number of drops used in the Raindrop. The 'Basic Recipe' that we teach in CARE suggests 3 drops per foot for the Foot VitaFlex and 4-6 drops on the back for each oil.

You can always reduce the number of drops to 1 per foot and 1 on the back. That will bring it to 24 drops. That is more appropriate for someone who is new to oils, healthy and does not have any 'Red Flags'.

- Lorrie Papach shared a great tip on how to reduce the chances of detoxing from Raindrop. She said, "I dilute with 50% grape seed oil, so there are likely no allergies [from the base oil]. I have an extra set of bottles and just fill them half and half, since I learned it doesn't lessen the effectiveness but lessens rapid detox. It is what I prefer."

When you follow this suggestion, just remember that base oil does go rancid in time. If you only do a Raindrop a few times a year, make sure you store these diluted oils in the fridge to reduce the chance of them going rancid.

- Do a half of a Raindrop. For this Receiver's first Raindrop, why can't you just do the Spinal VitaFlex on the feet and see how they respond. Perhaps you choose just to do a Raindrop on their back using 1-2 drops of each oil and skip the feet. This is one simple way to reduce the number of essential oils you apply to your Receiver.

Let's check out the characteristics of the oils again to give us a better idea of what oils are the 'heavy cleaners' of the group.

Oil	P, M or S
Valor	Monoterpenes & Sesquiterpenes
Oregano	Phenols
Thyme	Phenols
Basil	Phenols
Wintergreen	Phenols
Marjoram	Monoterpenes
Cypress	Monoterpenes & Sesquiterpenes
Peppermint	Phenols

You can see that five of the oils are the heavy cleaners. These are the oils that have a high concentration of phenols. Now, we do want to do some cleaning for sure; that is part of the beauty of Raindrop. You want to add some cleaners, but we want to certainly pull back on the amount of high phenolic oils used with someone who responds with a lot of 'red flag' answers.

Using these tips to reduce and/or dilute will do that. Just remember, the more toxins this Receiver has been exposed to, the less water they drink, and the less their exits are working means you want to reduce and dilute more.

Follow up!

You know how important it is that your Receiver drinks a lot of water to help eliminate those toxins that have been cleaned off. Give them water right away and educate them about the possible detoxing they may experience.

Sometimes we get so focused on the 'detoxing' possibilities that it is easy to forget discussing the benefits of Raindrop, which are SO many! Relaxed muscles, feeling grounded, feeling connected, immune support, reduce sore muscles, emotional release, etc.... Make sure you mention those too, along with detox indicators. We want people focused on all the good things that can occur from Raindrop.

If you give a Raindrop, then it is your responsibility to check in with your Receiver the next day. How are they feeling, are they drinking their water, and what other changes did they experience?

Getting their feedback on how they responded will help you determine the amount of essential oils you'll use for their next Raindrop.

If there is any detoxing going on, you can support them and remind them that when those toxins are eliminated if we don't add them back in, they are gone for good! Cleansing is a good thing!

It is also fun and rewarding to hear the positive and exciting comments. Usually, people comment about how they slept that night, they talk about how they felt emotionally or physically or how their time on the potty was very productive!

A Raindropper's Promise: "Thou Shall Not Skimp on Cypress or Valor®"

The two oils in the basic recipe that you don't want to reduce for any Receiver are Valor® blend and Cypress. There are a few reasons for that.

The first reason is Valor® and Cypress don't contain many phenols, so they will not add to the detoxing Raindrop provides. So, no worries about them contributing to overly detoxing Receivers.

Valor® is a balancing oil. It supports the Receiver by balancing them energetically and emotionally. We all need that, don't we? Valor® not only offers balance, but I was told it has the same frequency as bones so it also supports and assists the skeletal system to be balanced. When Valor® is used towards the end of Raindrop it is meant to help the Receiver hold any changes that they have experienced. I see Valor® as the glue to Raindrop.

As noted previously, Valor® has a base oil Caprylic/capric triglyceride. If someone is highly allergic to coconut, then use another oil that also offers emotional and energetic balancing, such as Believe® blend, Frankincense or Harmony® blend.

Cypress is mainly monoterpenes and sesquiterpenes. This essential oil supports the circulatory system. This includes the venous system and the lymphatic system.

The lymph system is a system that I get so excited about because it helps to remove toxins, large protein molecules, viruses and bacteria from our body. We always want this system to be supported and working well. We want it to be working extra well if someone will be detoxing. This is the system that will be 'taking out the trash' those phenol molecules are kicking up. It is the lymph system that will be responsible for eliminating the toxins released from the Raindrop. Cypress and citrus essential oils, staying hydrated and walking are three best ways to support the lymphatic system.

Chapter Three: Adding Other Oils

When I think of adding others oils into a Raindrop, I hear a line in my head from one of my daughter's favorite movies. In this movie, the teen heroine loves baking and while she is visiting her extended family in Paris, France, she learns the secret of 'je ne sais quoi' which in French mean 'I don't know what.' In a recipe, it is the special ingredient that is used to make a recipe unique and stand out. This 'je ne sais quoi' will not be the same each time the recipe is cooked or baked. The same is true for your Raindrops.

Why Would You Want To Add Other Oils To Raindrop?

We may add other oils if the client has a specific goal which can be addressed with an oil. This could be an emotional goal (to give clarity, bring joy or to be more present) or a physical goal (support digestive system, respiratory system or the brain). You may also get a nudge or feeling that a certain oil would complement the Raindrop and offer greater support for your Receiver.

What Oil and When?

There are a few ways you can determine what oil or oils to add:

1. **After the Trio**

    In C.A.R.E. Raindrop classes, we teach that you can add additional oils to support our client after the three oils we refer to as the 'Trio'; basil, wintergreen and marjoram are applied.

2. **"Why are you receiving this Raindrop Today?"**

    If you are asking or considering the eight questions I suggested in Chapter 2, question one is "Why are you receiving this Raindrop Today?"

    This question can often lead you right to the answer of what oils to add. If someone is looking for respiratory support, then you can add an oil that support the respiratory system such as Eucalyptus globulous, Raven® or R.C.® blend. If someone is looking for digestive support, then perhaps adding in Fennel or DiGize® blend would be appropriate.

If you don't know what oil will support the Receiver in their Raindrop goal, then take a look in your *Essential Oils Reference*. That will offer you many choices for your Receiver's goal.

Perhaps the support is emotional or simply to de-stress. What are some oils that would support that goal? Peace 'n Calming® blend, Stress Away® blend or Lavender are some that come to mind for me, how about you?

3. They Will Tell You

Many of my clients who are familiar with essential oils know right away what they want added. Some even bring their own oils with them.

If you are trading with or working with oily friends, then this may be the case.

4. Be Observant

Sometimes the Receiver may not know what would support them, or exactly what support they are looking for. Instead, they may tell you their story. Listen to their words, look at their posture and facial expression. That will give you so much information. You may hear in your head or heart or feel in your body the oils that would be a support for them.

One client who came to see me for Raindrop shared that her mom passed away six months ago and she felt that her heart was still heavy. The oils I pulled out of my kit to include in her Raindrop was Joy™ blend, Gentle Baby™ blend and Frankincense.

When I'm choosing an oil for emotional support, I usually don't tell the Receiver what oil I'm adding to the technique or that I'm even adding oils. I want their brain on relax mode, not trying to think of the rationality of why a particular oil was or was not chosen. At the end of the session, when they are dressed and drinking their water if they ask, then I'll share. Often they will say, "That was just the right oil or that was what I needed, thank you."

A few years ago, I had one client who oozed sadness. Her energy was low, her speech was slow, and her posture was slouched. She made Eeyore in Winnie the Pooh look like the life of the party. She was driving through town and wanted a Raindrop. She told me she "has had Raindrop before and it helped her back."

When I asked what her goal was in receiving this Raindrop, she didn't quite have an answer, but told me she was on this road trip to help her family.

I pulled out 3 oils for her to smell and see which one she was attracted to. Here are her replies when she smelled each oil.

Frankincense - "It smells okay."

Live My Passion® blend - "It's not bad."

Joy® blend - "This oil does not smell at all."

What? How could that oil not have a smell? Her frequency was SO LOW she didn't resonate at all with that high-frequency oil. You know which oil I chose to add her to Raindrop right, it was Joy® blend!

When she finished her Raindrop session with me, she was walking upright, there was a little twinkle in her eye again, and she said she was ready to continue her trip. I gave her a call the following day to check in and she told me all about the many sad and stressful events that were going on with her family in the past few months. Then she said that since her Raindrop, she felt lighter and better.

There is not just ONE WAY to choose an additional oil for your Receiver. The best advice I have for you is to listen to your Receiver, be observant of what is behind their words. Then listen to your own intuition, gut, and voice in your head or heart. This approach will never lead you wrong!

Chapter Four: Raindrop Is Just Like Cooking

When you are cooking, there are three reasons to replace ingredients called for in the recipe.

1. Sometimes, you need to replace ingredients because you are missing an ingredient. I often do this when I don't have milk called for in a muffin recipe; instead, I'll use yoghurt.

2. Another time, you may swap out an ingredient because of an allergy, like using almond milk instead of dairy milk.

3. The third reason to replace ingredients is to tailor your meal for a specific person's taste buds.

When You Are Missing an Oil

Sometimes, you may not have all the essential oils in the 'Basic Raindrop Recipe' because you ran out of the oil or it is out of stock. In my Raindrop career, Young Living was out of a few of the Raindrop oils. If I remember correctly, we were out of wintergreen at one point, cypress another time and Valor® for a (sad) long period. It happens when you are working with plants and working with a company that will not sell you something below their strict requirements.

This is not a time to panic and not do Raindrop, but a time to get creative and look at the possibilities of using other essential oils with a similar characteristic.

Recently, as Young Living was growing, they expanded into South Africa in September of 2019. They could not provide all of the oils immediately for distributors to purchase in South Africa.

One of the CARE Instructors put out the question and a list to the other instructors, "These are the oils they can get in South Africa. We can't get in oregano and basil yet. What oils would you use to replace oregano and basil for Raindrop?"

It was interesting to see the different ways that people approached this same question. I feel that people solve this problem based on their personalities. Some people are 'book' people, and others are 'gut' people. 'Book' people like to have the information to help them make a decision found in a book. To feel comfortable with their decision, the information they use needs to be found from a book, either in a chart, graph or paragraph. 'Gut' people don't necessarily need to find the information in the book but are comfortable with going by their intuition, gut feeling or past experience.

Either way of approaching which oil to use is fine and often leads to the same oils that are chosen. You choose which way you are comfortable with - it works, no worries!

When There Is an Allergy

The same is true for someone who says they have an allergy to an oil. When I first started using essential oils, I learned that you couldn't be allergic to pure essential oils because true essential oils don't contain protein molecules. You can read all about allergies and protein molecules in the *Chemistry of Essential Oils by Dr. David Stewart* Chap 12, Allergies.

As the years have passed and I've worked with more and more people, I have seen some unusual responses to essential oils. Are they allergies, emotional responses or detoxing? I'm not sure. One thing I am sure of is if someone tells me they are allergic to an oil, whether it is peppermint, wintergreen, or another oil, I will not argue with them. I'll share that it is protein molecules that we are allergic to, and pure essential oils do not contain proteins. I'll also share that the food additive or scents in candles are man-made molecules that we are allergic to and not the natural plant molecule we find in essential oils. Then I leave it in their hands. If they still are adamant that they are allergic to that oil, I will remove it from the Raindrop they will be receiving and replace it with another oil with a similar characteristic.

We know that intention and thought has a great deal to do with the outcome of our oils and Raindrop. I don't want my Receiver to experience their Raindrop with a fear that there is a small chance that they could have an allergic reaction to an oil being used. We don't want fear or worry to have a place in their Raindrop experience.

How to Choose a Replacement

If you are choosing a replacement oil for one out of stock or for one that someone is possibly allergic to, you can go about it the same way.

Let's use South Africa as an example. Here is a list of oils you could purchase from Young Living if you lived in South Africa in September 2019. If you notice, two important Raindrop oils are not on the list; oregano and basil.

Single Oils

1. Bergamot – 5ml
2. Cypress – 5ml
3. Eucalyptus Globulus – 5ml
4. Eucalyptus Radiata – 5ml
5. Frankincense – 5ml & 15ml
6. Geranium – 5ml
7. Grapefruit – 5ml & 15ml
8. Lavender – 5ml & 15ml
9. Lemon – 5ml & 15ml
10. Lemongrass – 5ml & 15ml
11. Myrrh – 5ml
12. Orange – 5ml & 15ml
13. Patchouli – 5ml
14. Cedarwood – 15ml
15. Citronella – 5ml
16. Clary Sage – 5ml
17. Copaiba – 5ml
18. Helichrysum – 5ml
19. Peppermint 5ml & 15ml
20. Rose – 5ml
21. Sacred Frankincense – 5ml
22. Spearmint – 5ml
23. Tea Tree – 5ml & 15ml
24. Wintergreen – 5ml
25. Ylang Ylang – 5ml
26. Vetiver – 5ml

Oil Blends

27. Christmas Spirit – 5ml
28. Citrus Fresh – 5ml & 15ml
29. Joy – 5ml
30. 12-month ER Loyalty Blend – 5ml
31. Melrose – 5ml
32. Peace & Calming – 5ml & 15ml
33. Purification – 5ml & 15ml
34. RC – 5ml & 15ml
35. Thieves – 5ml & 15ml
36. Raven – 5ml
37. Valor – 5ml & 15ml
38. White Angelica – 5ml
39. YL Haven (Stress Away) – 5ml & 15ml

Thanks to Evon McDonald for allowing me to share this list from her Face Book post.

Choosing a Replacement Oil

There are three ways that someone could approach choosing a replacement oil:

1. Using Chemistry
2. Using the EODR
3. Using the Oil's Characteristics

1. Using Chemistry

- Using *The Chemistry of Essential Oils*, look on page 498 to find the scientific name of oregano.

- Now turn to page 541 to look at Origanum compactum. We can see that oregano has 60-80% of phenols. We want to find an oil that has about that same amount.

- On page 571, there is a list of oils that have a high percentage of phenols. Choose an oil that you have that has a similar amount of phenols.

- Some of the choices are clove, fennel and basil.

"I try to sub an oil that is close or think about what my client needs. I always ask God to guide me in this and He always does."

Carol Bechtel

The upside to choosing an oil this way is that it was pretty quick and gives you a few possible oils to choose from.

The downside to choosing this way is that oils that have a large amount of the same constituent, like phenols, don't always support our bodies in the same way.

2. Using *the Essential Oil Desk Reference (EODR) 4th Edition*

- Let's take a look at how oregano can support us. You can find that on page 85 in the EODR.

- Under the 'Medical Properties' section, you'll see that oregano can support us in many ways. This allows us to tailor your Raindrop a bit. Is the Receiver looking for more immune support (antiviral and antibacterial properties) or more muscular support (anti-inflammatory properties)?

- Using the Personal Usage Reference section, look up your Receiver's goals. We'll say they want to support their immune system, so they don't get the cold going around the office. Look up 'Colds' on page 373.

- You'll see on page 373 you'll find some recommended oils for preventing colds.

- Choose one that you have.

3. Using the Oil's Characteristics

- Each oil used in the Raindrop Technique will support the body differently. Each oil supports a different body system, right?

- The oil that is missing, what does it support or what is its characteristic?

- The chart below gives you a real quick look at what system each oil supports.

- Oregano is a 'cleaner' and supports the immune system.

- What are other oils that do something similar? You may know right away, or you may need to look in the EODR for suggestions.

- Pick one that you have.

Oil	Supports
Valor	Balance Energies
Oregano	Immune System
Thyme	Immune System
Basil	Muscular System
Wintergreen	Skeletal System
Marjoram	Involuntary and Voluntary Muscles
Cypress	Circulatory and Lymph Systems
Peppermint	Digestive, Respiratory, Nervous Systems

By looking at our original example about the essential oils available in South Africa, which oil or blend would you use for oregano?

At some time, you'll need to find replacements for other oils not related to the Raindrop Technique. Now you have a path to a solution!

Tailor Your Raindrop to Fit That Person's Specific Needs

Once, I had planned a Chinese meal for dinner guests. I had rice, shrimp, carrots, onions, garlic, cashews and soy sauce ready to cook for our dinner.

Before dinner was cooked, we were chatting and nibbling on appetizers. My friend told me about how she had been on vacation and was sick for days! She had food poisoning after going to a Chinese restaurant, and she said, "I was SO sick; I don't think I will ever eat Chinese food again!"

Well, thankfully, I didn't choke on my appetizer. I excused myself and slipped back into the kitchen to look at my ingredients, which was:

Rice, shrimp, carrots, onion, cashews, garlic, and soy sauce.

After contemplating my ingredients for a few minutes, I created a new meal plan.

I replaced the cashews with cherry tomatoes and switched the soy sauce with fresh oregano and olive oil.

My Chinese stir fry transformed into an Italian Risotto, which I was so glad to hear was just what my dinner guest had been craving!

We can do the same 'ingredient swap' with our essential oils in the 'Basic Raindrop Recipe' to create a Raindrop that will support the Receiver's needs.

An example of this oil recipe swap is found in *Essential Oils Integrative Medical Guide*, on page 228. This wheel that Gary Young created gives us a wonderful quick guide to how we can tailor our Raindrops to support a very specific need of the Receiver.

I asked for permission to use a copy of that wheel in this resource guide, but I was told I could not, so instead, I'll describe it. The center of the wheel has three oils that are the 'hub' of Raindrop; Valor®, oregano and thyme. First, you need to balance with Valor®, then clean with oregano and thyme. The next oils chosen will replace the trio; basil, wintergreen, and marjoram. These replacements will be oils that are targeted for a certain system. Don't feel like you need to use all of the oils suggested. Use two to four of the oils that you have.

You may have noticed that you will not find cypress in the wheel, but I feel that this oil is a MUST to add to any Raindrop recipe. If you are 'cleaning' with oregano, thyme and other phenolic oils, you always want to support the lymphatic system with cypress.

So please, please, please always include cypress in your tailored Raindrop recipe.

I suggest you finish with the balancing blend, which is often Valor®. The effect of this oil is to help the body to hold changes, especially emotional and spinal alignment changes.

What if you don't have the oils listed in the wheel? What if you are looking to support your Receiver in a different way than what the wheel offers? Either way, simply look up in the EODR for the suggested oils for that goal and use two to four of those oils.

How cool is this? This concept now opens you up to countless Raindrop recipes specific to your Receiver's needs at that moment.

You can use the chart on the following page, 'System Supporting Raindrop', to help you create a tailored Raindrop.

Detoxing Considerations Still Apply

Remember, all the detoxing thoughts and advice in Chapter 2 still apply to these Tailored Raindrop Recipes. You can still give a very targeted Raindrop and reduce the oils you use. Perhaps you only do the Raindrop on the back and omit the feet. Again, the same thoughts apply. Ask questions and follow your intuition on the amount of oil used.

System Supporting Raindrop

This will follow the techniques and oil order used in CARE Raindrop Training.

> 1. Start your Raindrop like usual by balancing with Valor®.
> 2. Foot VitaFlex on the spinal points.
>   When doing the Foot VitaFlex you can use the Traditional Raindrop oils or use the replacements below.

3. On the back	4. Choose One System to Support These are suggestions.	5. Support the Lymph	6. Balance and Finish
Oregano **Thyme**	**Respiratory Support** Euc Glob Myrtle R.C.® Blend	**Cypress**	**Valor® and** **Peppermint**
Apply and Feather these as you typically do in Raindrop.	**Digestive Support** Fennel DiGize® Blend Peppermint	Follow with the usual techniques: Thumb VitaFlex, Finger Straddle, Stretch & Rock. Apply base oil and Palm Slide.	Apply these as you typically do, with Feathering and Arched Feather. Finish with moist heat pack.
	Skeletal Support Wintergreen PanAway® Blend		
	Immune Support Thieves® Blend Lemon Myrtle Euc Glob		
	Drop each System Supporting Oil and Feather, replacing Basil, Wintergreen and Marjoram. Continue with Finger Circles.		

Chapter Five: All About The Base

Did You Realize That You Can Tailor Your Raindrop Just By Changing Your Base Oil?

Yes, you sure can! I see the base oil choice, like icing on cupcakes. You can make the same vanilla cupcake, but once you change the icing flavor you now have a different cupcake.

A few icing flavor possibilities are vanilla, chocolate, strawberry or lemon. Each icing flavor will make that vanilla cupcake a bit different. You are simply tailoring your icing flavor to the taste buds of your birthday boy or girl!

The same is true for our Raindrops.

We normally use OrthoEase™ Massage Oil blend because it supports the muscles.

It is very common for people to replace OrthoEase™ with a base oil that does not contain any essential oils. That is normally done to reduce the number of essential oils the Receiver is exposed to and slow down the absorption of essential oils. This is often done to reduce detox.

In my practice, I work with many physically toxic clients, so I will often use safflower oil because I like how it feels for massage, and there is little chance for allergies. Other Raindroppers commonly use coconut, almond or Young Living's V-6™ blend.

Have you considered using some of the other massage blends that Young Living has?

In Adapting Raindrop Facebook group, we discussed this topic; here are what some of the members are doing. Look at how changing your base oil blend can tailor your Raindrop for your Receiver.

Marie Koepke, RN, shared that she uses Cel-lite Magic™ because it is a massage blend with oils that support lymph movement. If you are detoxing as you do with Raindrop, you certainly want that lymph system supported. Such a brilliant adaptation!

Lorrie Papach said she uses OrthoSport™ for her son, a wrestler. He benefits from using OrthoSport™, which is blended to support active, sore muscles.

Maximilian Gasseholm was newlywed when this topic came up, so it was no surprise he thought of using Sensation™ massage oil! What a great idea for Valentine's or date night.

Tabatha Hubbard commented that she gave a modified Raindrop to her 4 yr old and used Seedlings™ Baby Oil, which made a great base oil.

Relaxation™ Massage Oil is a great option for those who are looking for relaxation and a total 'chill' experience during their Raindrop session.

Dragon Time™ massage oil is perfect for women working on balancing their hormones.

I hope this gives you an idea of how to tailor your Raindrops by simply switching your base oil massage blend choice!

Chapter Six: Just Give 'Em A Quickie!

When people find out that my husband and I are Massage Therapists, they often say the same thing with a dreamy look in their eye, "Oh, you are *SO* lucky! You must give each other massages ALL the time. That is amazing; I wish my husband/wife would give me massages!"

After we hear that statement, we just laugh and laugh and then ask them if they ever heard of the story of The Shoemaker's Children. Basically, the story is about how the shoemaker's children run around with shoes that are too small and full of holes because the last thing he wants to do when he gets home is make shoes for his kids.

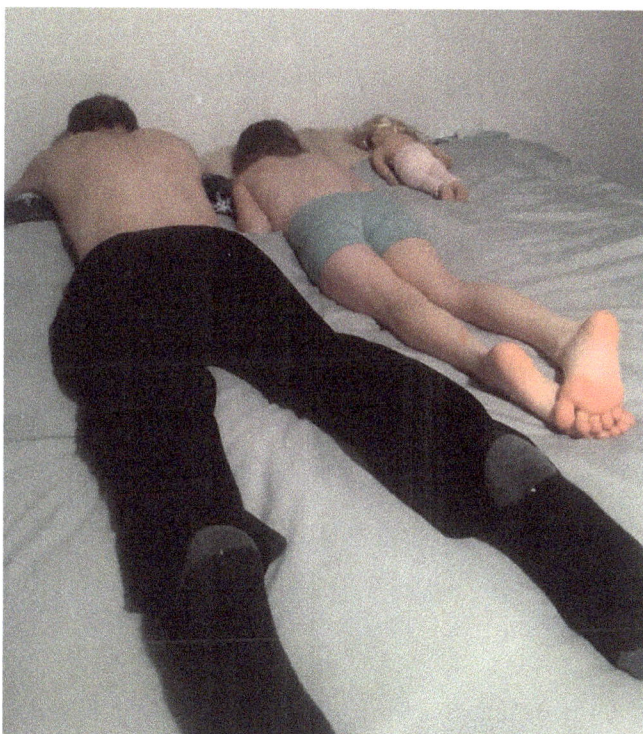

Unfortunately, we are the same way. We are at the office working on clients all day, and honestly, when I get home, I really don't want to give my hubby a full hour massage. I have other things I want to do or have to do at home. He can't be mad I'm sharing this with you because I know he feels exactly the same way!

We work on each other now and then when we are dealing with an ache or pain, but we really give each other 'Quickies'. That is our silly joke, but I'm all for Quickies and encourage you to be open to Quickies.

You might not be a Massage Therapist and roll your eyes when your spouse asks you to massage their neck, but I know you are busy. You don't always have the TIME to do a full hour, fancy Raindrop that you experienced in a Raindrop class or that your Massage Therapist or Raindrop Practitioner would do for you. What you do have time for are Quickies.

I want you to be able to give a Raindrop to your family when they need it, so they can receive the benefits right there and then. Don't guilt yourself over the fact that it is a Quickie; just get it done.

When you give a Quickie, you will use the tips I share in Chapter 7, *Giving a Raindrop When You Don't Have a Massage Table*. The goal here is to get those oils on and tailor the oils used based on what would benefit your Receiver at that time (Part 1 of this Resource Guide).

Maybe you'll do just Foot VitaFlex on the spinal points of the feet; maybe you'll just apply the oils on the back. Perhaps you'll do both without all the extra techniques typically used in Raindrop; you just feather in the oils after you drop them. The choice is up to you, based on how much time you have, how much sleep you've had in the past 24 hours and how long your Receiver is going to lay there.

The biggest takeaway I want you to get from this chapter is that it is OKAY to be flexible with this technique. Life is busy and crazy. Let's use the philosophy behind Raindrop and harness the power of our 'essential oil subway system', our nervous system, to get those oils on and in our family to support their health.

During flu season, I'll routinely round up my family and have them lay on the bed for a Quickie Raindrop. I took this picture right before I started dropping oils on their back. Each time I dropped an oil, I explained to my daughter why I chose the oil. She is becoming quite the educated oiler! What I missed in this picture is what happened after giving them their Quickies. My girl said she wanted to give ME my Raindrop! So with her Dad's supervision, she gave me my 'Quickie Raindrop'. As she dropped each oil and feathered them in, she told me how each one supports my body to stay healthy.

I love this memory and am proud of our little family that we were flexible and took advantage of this teachable moment. I hope this story inspires you to be adaptable and open to 'Quickie Raindrops' for your family.

Part 2

Comfort of the Receiver

Chapter Seven: Giving Raindrop When You Don't Have A Massage Table

Maybe you don't have a massage table yet. Perhaps you don't have the room to store one or set one up. I don't want you to feel like you cannot give Raindrops to your family because you don't have a massage table. There are so many options that offer you the opportunity to give a relaxing and enjoyable Raindrop experience to friends and family, even if you don't have a massage table. You can certainly make a few adaptations, and I will show them to you in this chapter.

Don't feel like you have to skip doing VitaFlex spinal points on the feet if you don't have a massage table. I'll show you a simple adaptation to this technique without using a massage table.

For each *Don't Have a Massage Table* option, I'll explain the pros and cons. I'll share tips to make these adaptations comfortable and cozy for your Receiver and comfortable for the Giver.

Since a picture is worth a thousand words, I have quite a few for you to look at in this chapter. I also have videos showing these techniques too. You can request access to these videos by going to https://adaptingraindrop.com/oilyfamvideos/

You'll find a 'Notes Page' in this book that correlates to each video. I added these intending to give you a place to take notes as you watch the videos. You also can use these note pages to jot down what works best for your family and friends. You can then refer back to your notes and thoughts whenever you need them.

Foot Vitaflex without a Massage Table

When you are giving a Raindrop to someone who will not be lying on a massage table, you will need to adapt your Foot VitaFlex on the Spinal Points of the feet.

You can use this adaptation anytime you want to do some VitaFlex on someone's foot. This method can be used when giving Raindrop to pregnant mothers, anyone who cannot lay on their backs for a long period, a Receiver who is unable to get on a massage table or when you are doing Raindrop at the Kitchen Table.

If your Receiver is sitting on a chair, you can simply sit on the floor and access their feet. This works perfectly for VitaFlexing the spinal points on the feet.

Your Posture

(Picture #1)

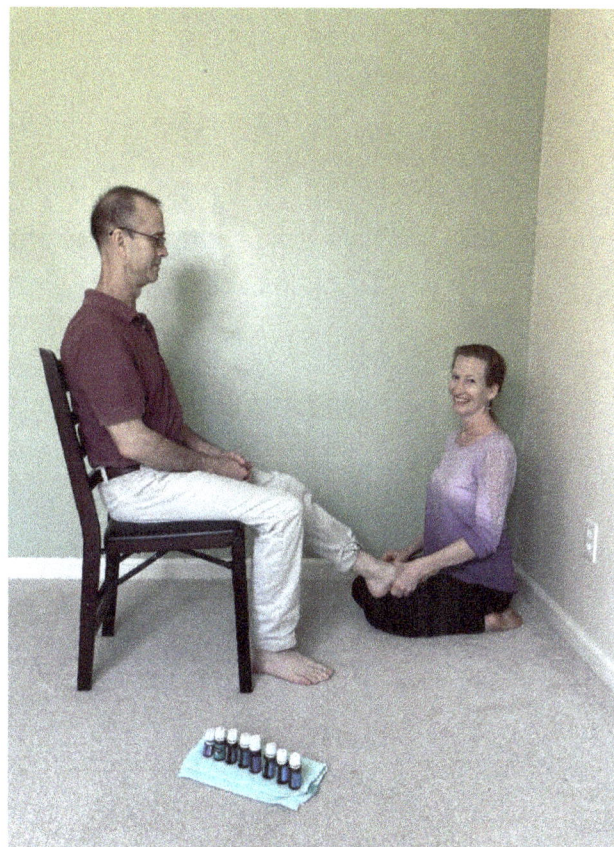

This sounds easy enough, but depending on what your Receiver is sitting on, say a chair, couch or bed, that will affect their foot height. The height of your Receiver's foot will affect your posture. It is important that while doing foot VitaFlex, your posture is correct. Your posture will either make this time pleasant, or a *'my neck and shoulder are hurting, let's get this done* quickly*'* experience for you. Your posture will also affect the VitaFlex technique. If you are in good posture and comfortable, you'll do a much better job.

To see if you are in good posture or need to make adjustments to your positioning, look at your shoulders while you are doing foot VitaFlex. If your shoulder is not raised or lowered, that is the perfect height of the Receiver's foot. (Picture #1)

If you find that when doing Foot VitFlex, the shoulder of your VitaFlexing arm is rising to your ear that means your Receiver's foot is too high for you. (Picture #2)

When this happens, place your Receiver's foot on the floor instead of your lap. When you lower the Receiver's foot, you'll notice that your shoulder should drop. Your neck will thank you for this better posture.

What if you, as the Giver, are not too comfortable getting down on the floor? No worries, you can still offer Foot VitaFlex to your Receiver without issue. Use a chair along with a stool. I like the adjustable rolling chair because it gives me the ability to move around easily, it also gives the chance to raise or lower MY body to put the Receiver's foot in a comfortable location for me to work on.

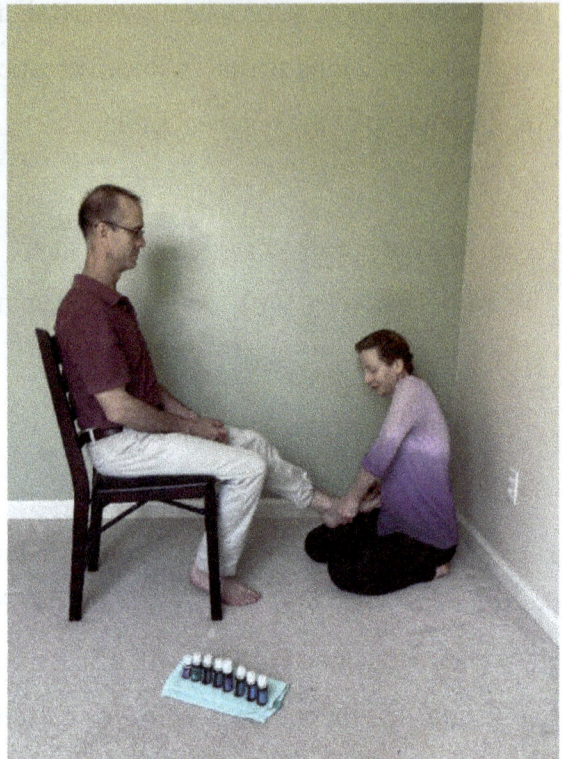

With the Receiver and Giver sitting in chairs, you'll just need a stool for the Receiver's foot to be propped up on. With your adjustable chair, you can adjust the height of your chair to get your Receiver's foot in a comfortable location for your body.

If you don't have an adjustable chair, you can also place your Receiver's foot on a pillow to raise it.

The goal is to have both the Giver and Receiver comfortable. As the Giver, you need to pay attention to your shoulders. They should not be raised up to your ears while giving Foot VitaFlex. You may very likely get a sore back, shoulder, and/or neck if that happens. (Picture #3)

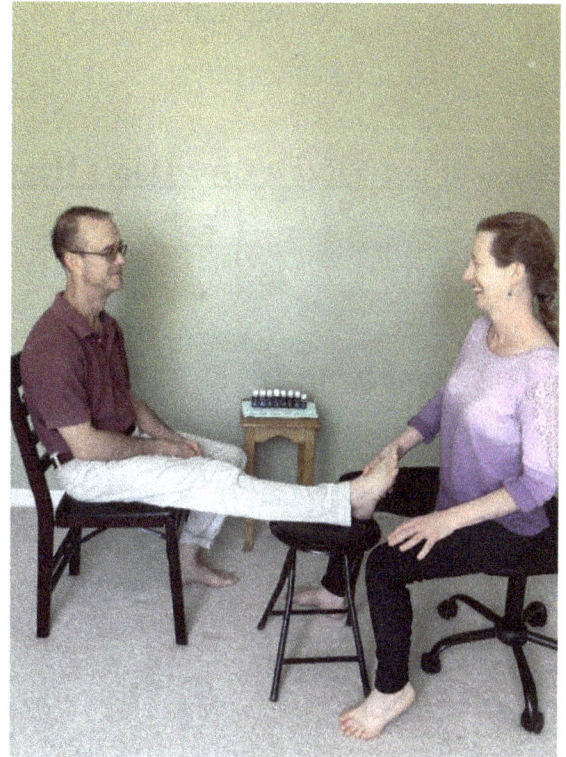

Keeping your shoulder in neutral will help keep you comfortable, give a better VitaFlex and be more attentive to your Receiver's needs.

When you switch to the other foot, you'll also need to switch your VitaFlex hand. This is where having a rolling chair is convenient. You can just roll on over to the other foot. Like in traditional Raindrop, you'll need to switch your VitaFlex hand when you switch feet. (Picture #4)

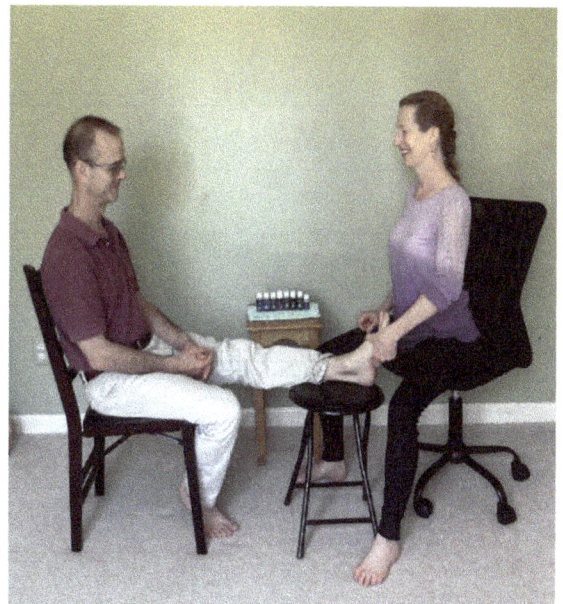

Notes Page:

To watch this video on these adaptations, just request a link to the videos here: https://adaptingraindrop.com/oilyfamvideos/

Foot VitaFlex for Don't Have a Massage Table Options

Tips:

- Adjust your height based on the Receiver's height.
- Is your shoulder moving up? Receiver's foot needs to be lowered or Giver needs to be raised up.

Notes:

_____

_____

_____

_____

_____

_____

_____

_____

_____

Raindrop on the Floor

One of the benefits of giving Raindrop to your Receiver on the floor is that it is inexpensive and easy.

The cons are that this can be quite uncomfortable for both the Receiver and Giver due to posture.

(Picture #5)

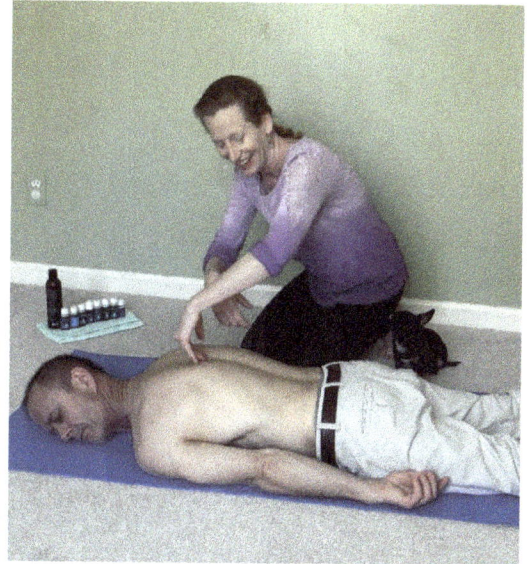

If you look at picture #5, the Receiver is lying on the floor with their head turned to the side. After a while, this can become very uncomfortable, and your Receiver will most likely want to turn their head to the other side because their neck is getting stiff.

(Picture #6)

Also, when the Receiver's head is turned to the side, it does not allow you to feather up to the occipitals or base of the skull. It is important to make sure you feather up the neck and to the base of the skull, where the cranial nerves exit.

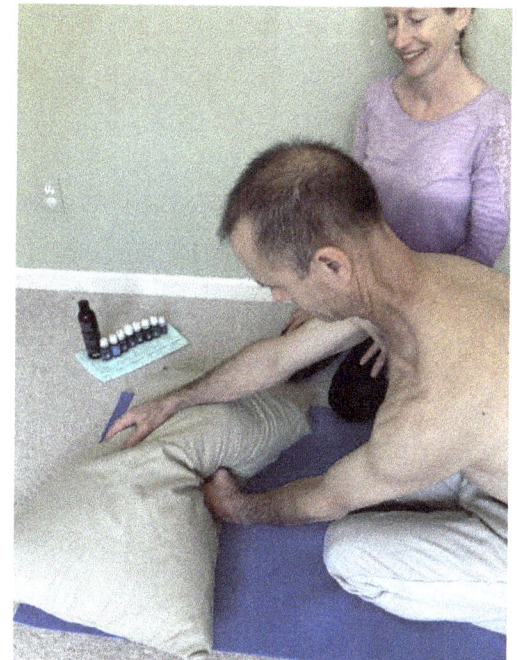

The cranial nerves are important to incorporate in Raindrop because these nerves are the ones that travel to and support the senses found in the head. The base of the skull is where the cranial nerves exit, which then innervates the head. You can't forget the Vegas nerve, also known as 'The Wanderer' This nerve has many jobs, including relaxation and supporting many of our organs.

To ensure you get the neck and base of the Receiver's skull as they are laying on the floor, use a large pillow and punch it into a 'V' shape. (Picture #6)

Position the pillow, so the point is at the top; this is where the Receiver's forehead will lay. The opening of the 'V' is now facing them, and this creates the space for the Receiver's nose and mouth to be so that breathing is possible, as in picture #7.

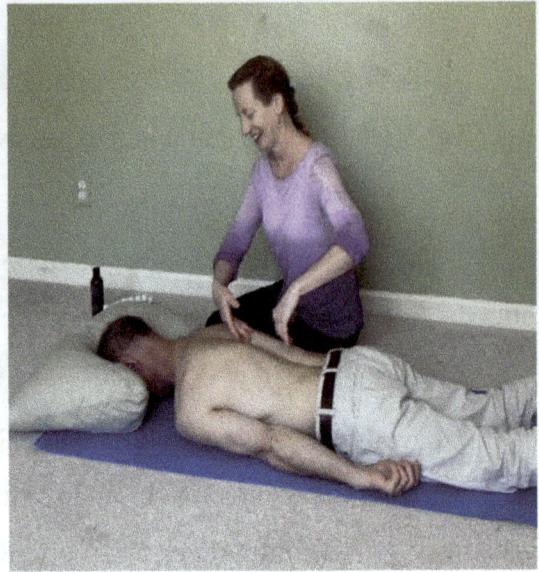

(Picture #8)

If your Receiver still feels like they need more space for their face to lay, then they can use their arms to prop up their head a bit more. (Picture #8)

To keep your Receiver as comfortable as possible, use a mat or blanket for them to lay on. Don't forget to use sheets or blankets on top to keep them warm and cozy.

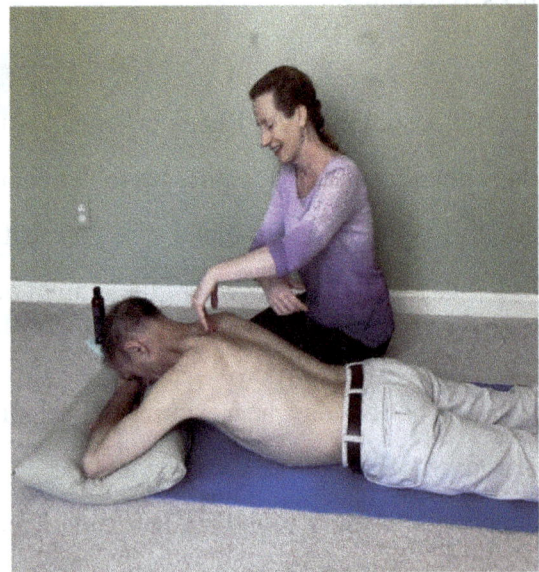

With your Receiver on the floor like this, it allows you to do all the techniques typically used on the back. One caution for you is to remember that the neck is not supported, so don't put pressure on the cervical spine or neck. While you are on the floor, you'll find that to do all of the techniques on the back, like Thumb VitaFlex and Finger Circles, you'll be moving around and repositioning your body a lot!

When it comes time for the moist heat pack, you'll apply and remove it the same way as if your Receiver was on a massage table.

Notes Page:

To watch this video on these adaptations, just request a link to the videos here: https://adaptingraindrop.com/oilyfamvideos/.

Option 1: On the Floor

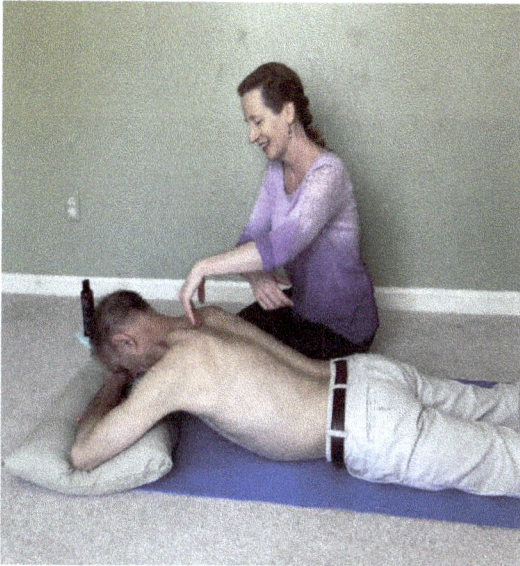

Pros:

- Fast, inexpensive, good for quick Raindrops.

Cons:

- Uncomfortable for both Giver and Receiver.
- Poor neck alignment.

Tips:

- Pillow punched into a 'V' for nose and mouth.
- Use arms to give more space for nose to allow for better breathing.

Notes:

_____

_____

_____

_____

_____

_____

_____

_____

_____

Raindrop on a Bed

Another option similar to giving Raindrop on the floor is giving Raindrop on a bed.

If you are going to do Foot VitaFlex, you can do that with your Receiver sitting on the edge of the bed as described in *Foot VitaFlex without a Massage Table*. If you don't have a lot of time or the attention span of your Receiver is short, you can always consider skipping the feet and moving right on to the back!

(Picture #9)

Raindrop on a bed is a good option because it offers our Receiver a soft, comfortable place to lay. Once they have their Raindrop and the moist heat pack is removed, they can just stay snuggled up and take a nap! This is a perfect option for family members when they are sick, and you are giving them Raindrops to support their immune system.

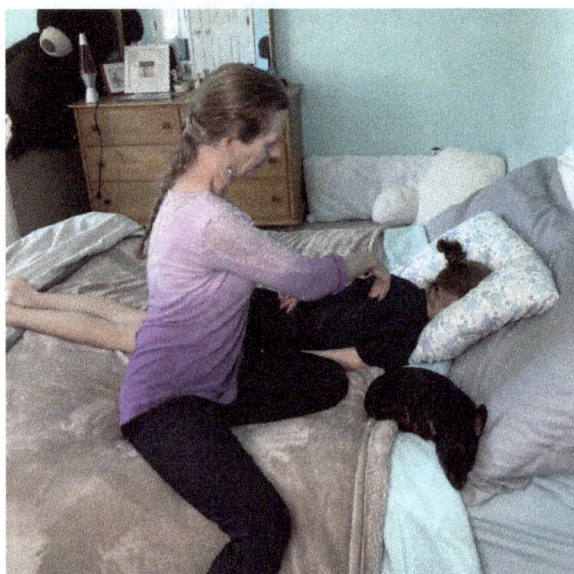

The only drawback for the Receiver is that their head is turned to the side, which does not give you access to their neck. You can use the same 'punch a pillow' tip used in *Raindrop on the Floor*. This creates a 'V' shape which allows support for the forehead and space for your Receiver's nose for breathing. (Picture #9)

If they need more space for their nose, they can rest their head on their forearms. If giving a Respiratory Supporting Raindrop, make sure you do all the techniques up to the occipital ridge or base of the skull. The cranial nerves exit from the base of the skull, and it is these nerves that support the sinuses.

(Picture #10)

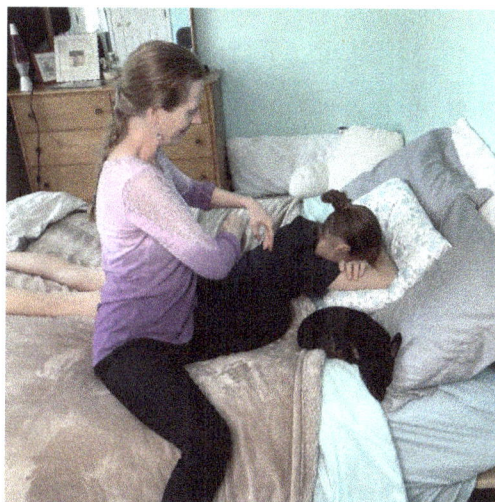

As the Giver, you can sit at the side of the bed like in picture #10, but you'll find that you'll need to do a lot of twisting at the waist and stretching. It is not easy to move around in this position.

(Picture #11)

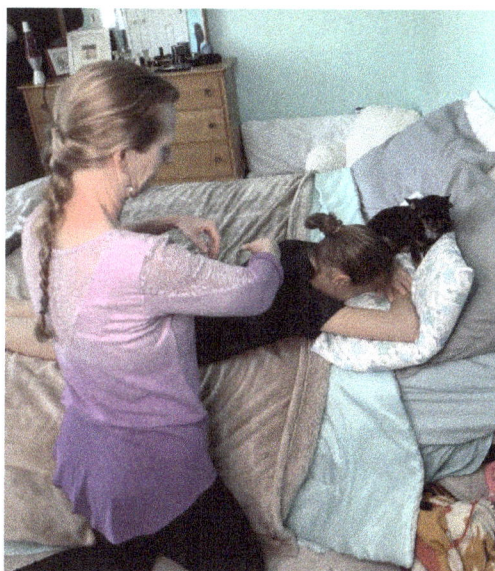

To help you feel more comfortable and give you more movement, have your Receiver move to the edge of the bed, and you work on your knees. (Picture #11)

Working on your knees allows you to walk on your knees from sacrum to head vs leaning over like you did when sitting on the side of the bed. This works best on lower beds that are typically used for little guys.

Another option is to use a small stool or rolling chair with your Receiver lying parallel to the edge of the bed. This saves your knees and gives you more stability than sitting on the side of a soft bed. With a rolling chair, you'll have the added fun rolling from hip to head instead of stretching or walking on your knees.

Applying the heat pack would be the same as typically done on a massage table. The best part is that your Receiver does not have to get up; they can just roll over and nap like my daughter does in picture #12.

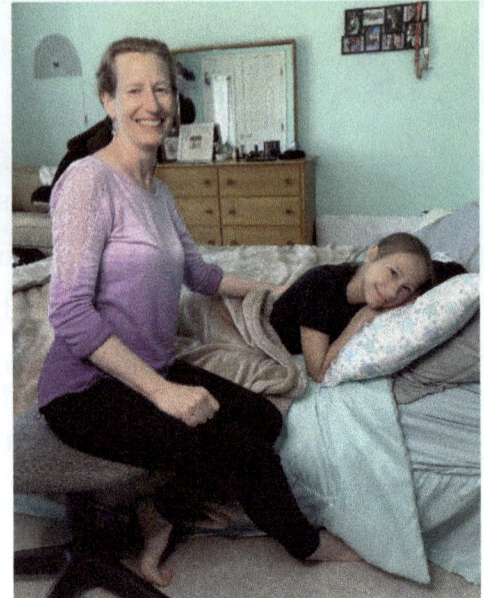

Notes Page:

To watch this video on these adaptations, just request a link to the videos here: https://adaptingraindrop.com/oilyfamvideos/

Option 2: On a Bed

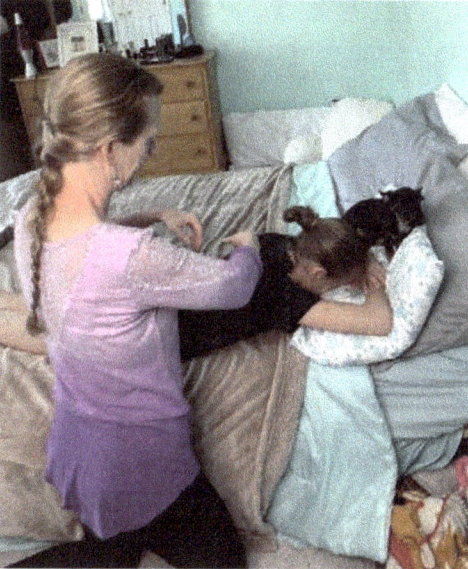

Pros:

- Fast, inexpensive, and everyone has one; good for 'Quickie Raindrops'.

Cons:

- Uncomfortable for both Giver and Receiver.
- Poor neck alignment.

Tips:

- Pillow punched into a 'V' for nose and mouth.
- Use arms to give more space for nose to allow for better breathing.

Notes:

_____

_____

_____

_____

_____

_____

_____

_____

_____

_____

Raindrop at the Kitchen Table

You might think I'm crazy for suggesting this, but hear me out. Once you see how comfortable both you and the Receiver can be using this adaptation, you will love giving Raindrop at the kitchen table. Don't worry; I didn't say ON the kitchen table. We will not lay down on the kitchen table as if it was a massage table. Nope, we are doing Raindrop AT the kitchen table.

The pros to this method are that you will be standing the whole time as the Giver. You will not be bent at weird angles that can cause your back to hurt. Depending on how many pillows and blankets you use, you can make your Receiver super comfortable, so comfortable that they may fall asleep!

Honestly, I have not found a con to this adaptation.

This technique is great for pregnant moms or anyone else who can't lay on their tummy. It is a perfect way to give Raindrop to Receivers who can't physically get on a massage table. It also is perfect for families who want to give a full Raindrop but don't have a massage table.

(Picture #13)

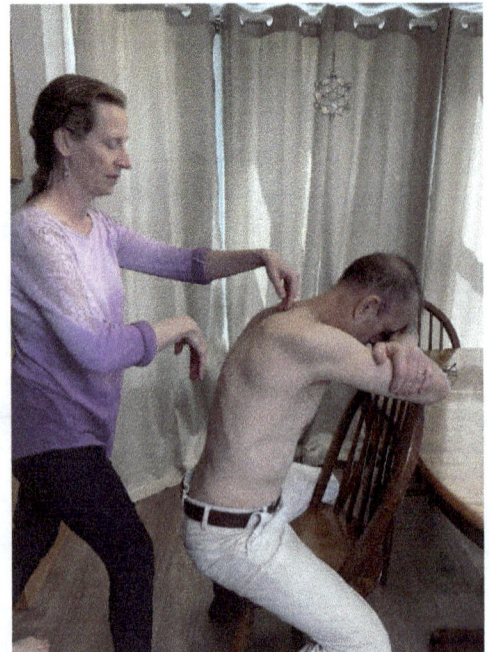

In my practice, I've used this method for pregnant moms, a client who broke her ribs and could not lay down due to pain and a senior who could not just 'hop up' onto a massage table and flip over from back to stomach.

We'll start with the most basic and simple option, which is also the least comfortable. Then, I'll explain how simple changes can make things cozier for your Receiver.

The first adaptation is to turn a kitchen chair around and have your Receiver straddle it backwards as if they were riding a horse. From there, they can lean their arms on the back of the chair. You now have full access to their back. (Picture #13)

You can easily do all the oil application and feathering from sacrum to occipitals without a problem. Since your Receiver's chest is not supported, you don't want to put a lot of pressure on their back when doing techniques typically used in Raindrop like Finger Circles and Thumb VitaFlex.

(Picture #14)

To improve this adaptation, you can place a pillow on the back of the chair for your Receiver to lean their arms on, as shown in picture #14.

If you are working with women or want to keep your Receiver warmer, then have them put on a button-down shirt backwards. This allows access to their spine while giving them more modesty and warmth.

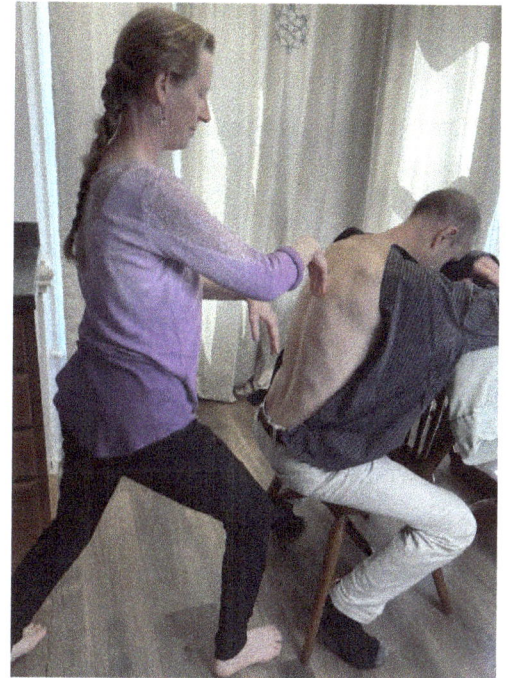

Here are the additional adaptations to make *Raindrop at the Kitchen Table* a truly warm, cozy experience.

We'll start by switching out the kitchen chair for a stool, so there is no chair back to deal with. Push the stool close to the kitchen table and stack a few pillows on the table. Propping up pillows will 'raise' the table and allow the Receiver to lean on to the pile of soft pillows with their upper chest and head. They should use their arms to 'hug on to' the pillows for additional support. You have the flexibility now to make your pile of pillows as high as necessary to keep your Receiver comfortable.

You can also take one pillow, placing it half on the table and half off it. This will allow your Receiver to lay their upper chest and belly on it and the table. This gives more support to their chest so you can safely apply pressure with Finger Circles and other techniques. (Picture #15)

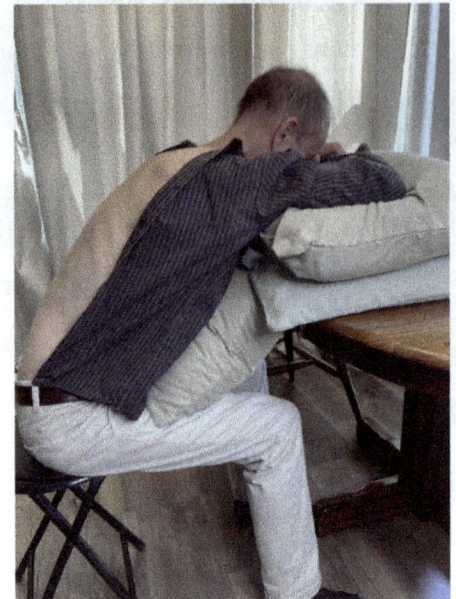

When you are dropping oils, gravity will play a role—no pun intended! You'll notice how quickly those drops of oil travel down, down, down. To ensure the oils don't go farther than the 'no-fly zone', you'll need to do two things. The first is to drop your oils higher up than usual. Drop the oils on the spine, but don't drop them any lower than that between the shoulder blades.

The next thing you'll need to do is quickly get to your first set of feather strokes. This will stop the oils from rolling south. The rest of your feathering for that oil does not need to be done faster than usual.

(Picture #16)

When your Receiver is sitting on a stool that allows you to get close to their back to do more than just the feathering techniques, with your Receiver's chest supported with the table and pillow, you can now do all the techniques that are typically used in Raindrop. You'll just need to make a few simple adaptations.

Finger Circles:

You can do Finger Circles, just like when your Receiver is lying face down on a massage table. The only change you'll need to make is your posture. You'll need to lower your body to do this technique on their lower back. To make your body lower, you simply need a wide stance. (Picture #16)

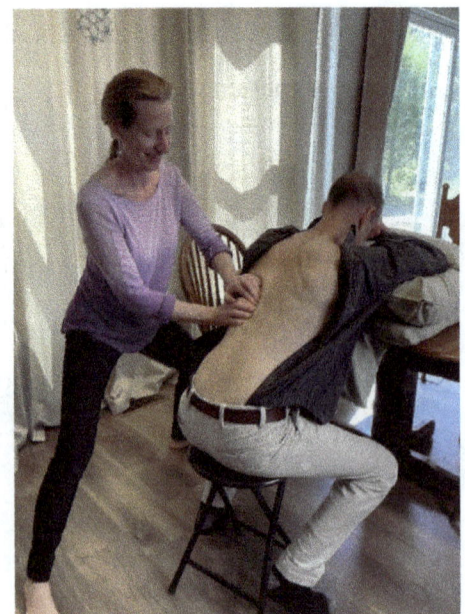

Stretch and Rock:

You will not be able to get as much of a stretch as when a Receiver is lying on a massage table, but you can still do some. Again, the key to doing this technique when your Receiver is at the kitchen table is you need a low and wide stance. It will allow you to have more strength in your stretch than if you are bending at the waist. (Picture #17)

Avoid stretching the neck or cervical spine in this position since the neck is bent and not in alignment with the spine.

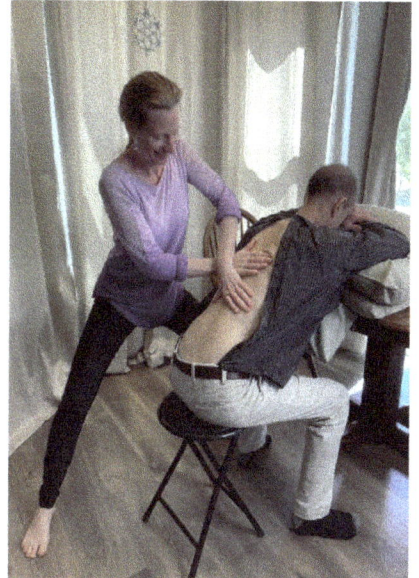

(Picture #18)

Saw Maneuver:

The Saw Maneuver can be done from low back to the top of the cervical spine. You will notice that their body does not rock much. The adaptation you will make as the Giver is standing with a wide stance to protect your back. (Picture #18)

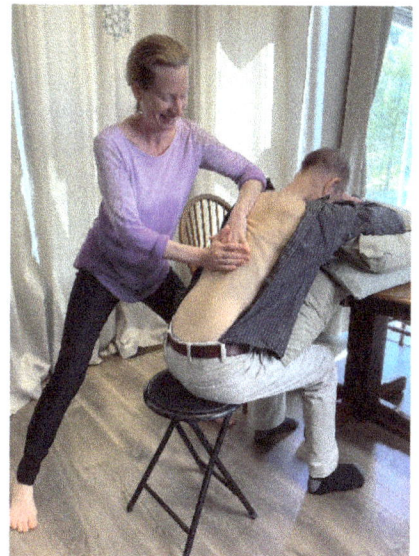

Palm Slide:

This will be done the same way as if you were doing this technique to a Receiver on a massage table. Once again, the key to your strength and keeping your back from not complaining is a wide stance. (Picture #19)

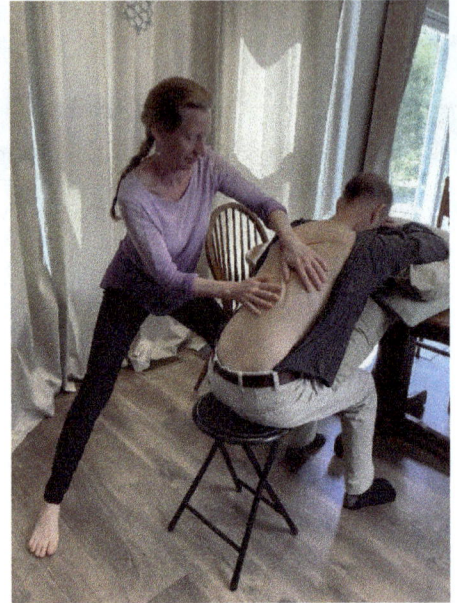

(Picture #20)

Moist Heat Pack:

At this point, you will make quite a few changes when applying the moist heat pack. To help the towels stay put and not slide down, place some of the dry towels over your Receiver's shoulders. If you use one dry towel and fold it over to make a 'hot pack sandwich', make the fold by the sacrum. This will stop the moist towel from slipping out. (Picture #20)

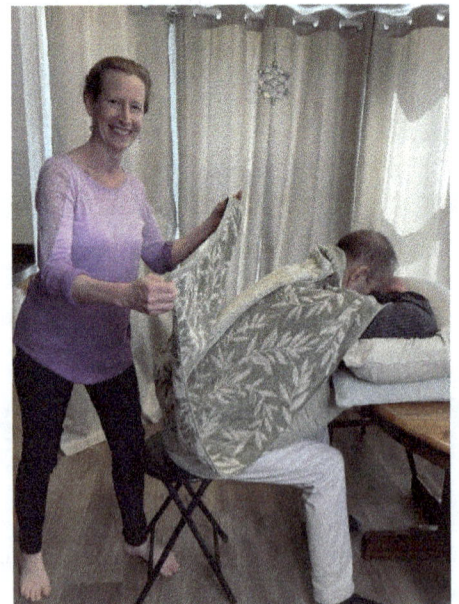

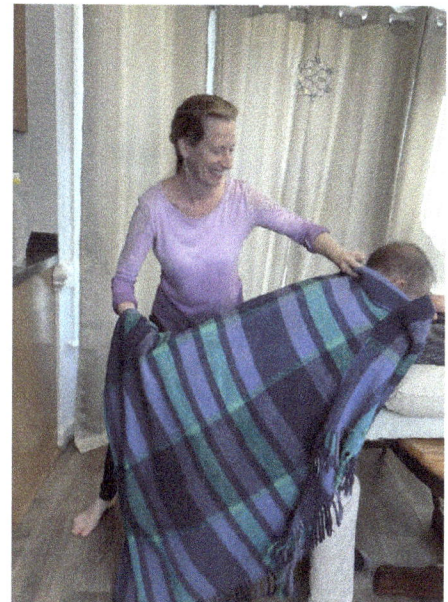

To keep your Receiver warm and comfortable while they 'cook', you can cover them with a sheet, blanket or both. (Picture #21)

(Picture #22)

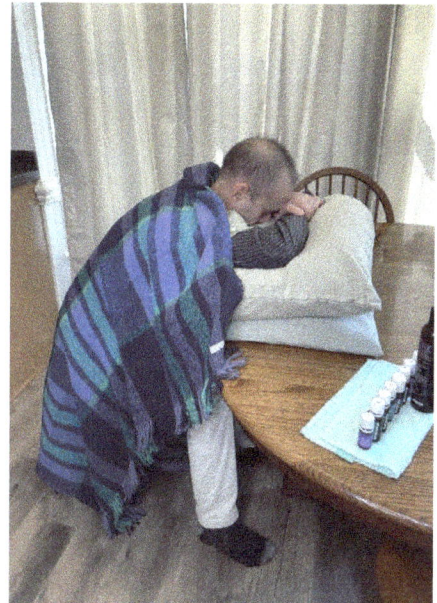

Taking off the towel will be different then what you learned for a Receiver on a massage table. Here, we are going to use gravity to help us! First, hold the sheet and/or blanket by your Receiver's shoulder to keep them in place. Slide your other hand under the blanket from the side and grab hold of the moist heat pack sandwich laying on their low back or sacrum. To remove the moist heat pack, simply pull down. It will quickly fall; you just need to guide it out of the blanket tent. (Picture #22)

Your Receiver is still covered and warm; they are toasty and comfortable. At this time, they can relax for as long as they'd like. A benefit to this technique is that your Receiver can stand up from the stool. They do not need to hop off a massage table. Once they are ready, they can easily wrap themselves up in the sheet or blanket and move to a private room to change.

A tool that I found recently is a blow-up airplane pillow, which replaces all the pillows I used. It is quick to inflate, very small, and easy to store when deflated. I like how versatile it is; just changing the position of the airplane pillow, I can use it with an adult or a child. (Picture #23 & #24)

(Picture #23)

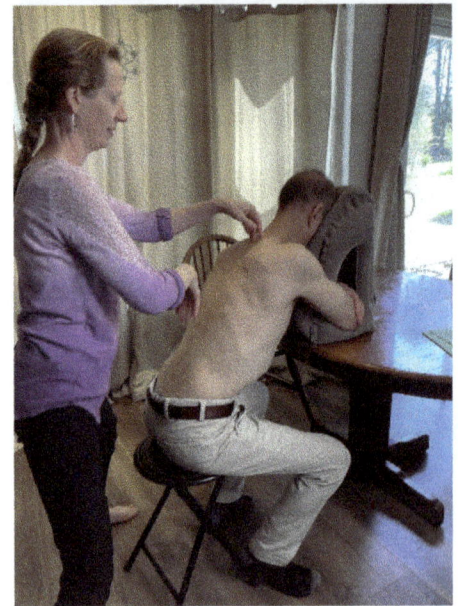

The only con to this tool is that you cannot clean it well. You might consider using a thin washable cloth towel or paper towel on the inflatable pillow to keep it clean.

(Picture #24)

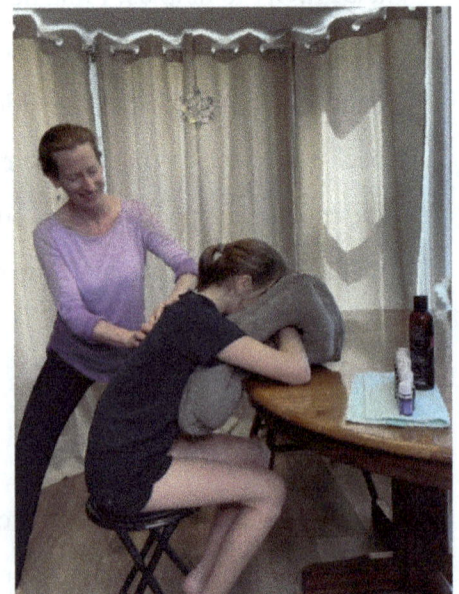

Using these adaptations and tools, you can give a comfortable Raindrop to the whole family at your kitchen table! You'll find links to the stool and inflatable pillow in my Tools Page at www.AdaptingRaindrop.com if you want to purchase them.

Notes Page:

To watch this video on these adaptations, just request a link to the videos here: https://adaptingraindrop.com/oilyfamvideos/

Option 3: At the Kitchen Table

Pros:

- Good for Receivers who cannot lay on massage table.
- Comfortable for Receiver (with tips!)
- Good posture for Giver.
- Easy set up.
- Can do all techniques when upper chest is supported.

Cons:

- Little pressure on back if upper chest is not supported.

Tips:

- Drop oils high up on spine.
- Button down shirt on backwards for females.
- Use many pillows or airplane pillow.
- Use stool instead of chair
- Pull moist heat pack from bottom.

Notes:

_____

_____

_____

_____

_____

_____

_____

_____

_____

_____

Chapter Eight: Keeping Your Receiver Comfortable on a Massage Table

While we are doing Raindrops, we want our Receivers to be as comfortable as possible while they are on a massage table. Sometimes there are complaints, and it is a horrible feeling when you don't know what to do to relieve what is causing discomfort to your Receiver.

The most common complaint from Receivers is that their sinuses get stuffy from lying face down. I'll show you how to remedy that. Some of the members of Adapting Raindrop will also share their Stuffy Sinuses tips with you.

When Your Receiver Has Stuffy Sinuses from Lying Face Down On a Massage Table

There is no doubt about it; they invariably get a stuffy nose when people lay face down for a long period. For most people, this is a slight annoyance, but for others, this can cause discomfort and frustration. Putting a moist heat pack on your Receiver at the end of their Raindrop experience is a calming, relaxing and enjoyable experience. If their sinuses are full and uncomfortable, then lying face down with the hot pack for an additional ten minutes may be more torturous than enjoyable for them.

In this chapter, I'll share how to check in with your Receiver to see if they are in a silent face down misery or would be content staying in this position for an additional ten minutes.

You'll also learn how to transition your Receiver to lying face up and lying on the moist heat pack.

I also have some great tips on preventing stuffy sinus discomfort from Raindroppers in Adapting Raindrop.

Just Ask Them:

Sometimes our Receivers can be very vocal about the discomfort they are experiencing, and other times they keep it quiet. When you get to the moist heat pack part of Raindrop, I find the easiest thing to do is ask a simple question.

"The last part of this Raindrop is a moist heat pack applied to your back. Would you like to stay face down for the moist heat pack for another ten minutes, or would you prefer to flip over one more time to lay face up?"

You asked them, so the decision is all theirs. You don't need to worry or guess.

I find that most Receivers are very content lying face down, and they have no desire to change their position. Those Receivers that are uncomfortable will jump at this opportunity to lay on their back again, even if it means one more flip on the table and some adjusting.

Flip them Over:

(Picture #25)

If your Receiver chooses to lay on their back for the moist heat pack, then the first thing you'll need to do is assist them in turning over.

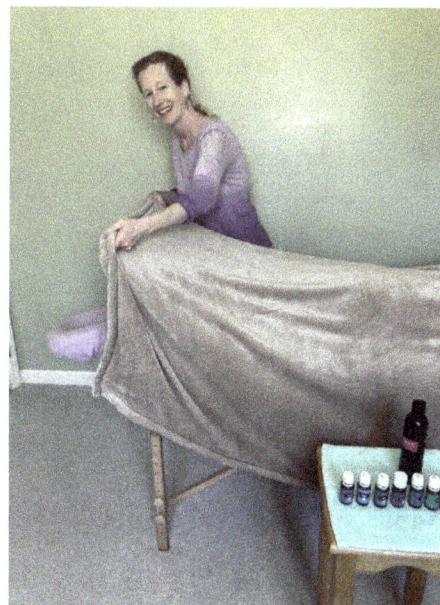

When a Receiver flips over from their stomach to back, it is always helpful to:

- Hold up the sheet just a few inches, so they don't get tangled in the sheet while flipping.
- Ask them to 'scoot down' before flipping over. This allows them to have their head on the massage table instead of the cradle after flipping over. You'll notice in picture #25 that I can't even see my Receiver on the

63

table after they scooted down a bit. This way, they will stay toasty warm and covered too.

Once that is done, and they are now laying face up, you'll need to get your dry towel and hot moist towel to make the moist heat pack sandwich.

(Picture #26)

Sitting Up:

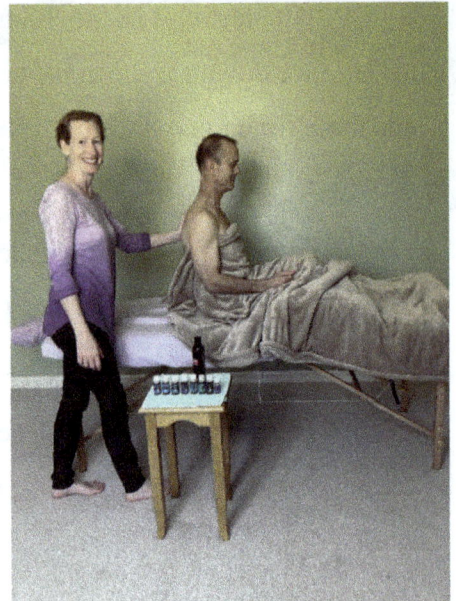

There are two ways you can coach your Receiver to move so you can position the moist heat pack for them to lay on.

The first option is to coach your Receiver to simply sit up. Before your Receiver sits up, ask them to take their arms out from under the sheets. This will allow them to keep that sheet close to their body when sitting up for a few minutes. (Picture #26)

(Picture #27)

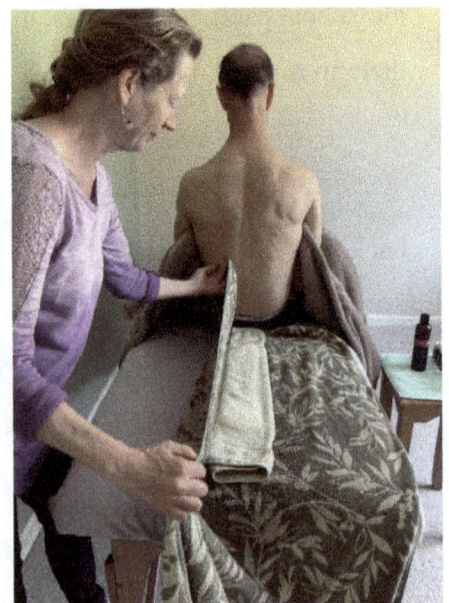

A tip to make sitting up from a lying position easier is to ask your Receiver to bend their knees first. If you are strong enough and have a sturdy back, you can also offer your arm for assistance in pulling up.

Once your Receiver is sitting up, you have access to the table and their back. You can easily lay out the dry towel, then the moist heat pack in the middle and finish with the dry towel on top. When you lay out the moist heat pack sandwich, start it right at your Receiver's sacrum. (Picture #27)

Stand at the head of the massage table and check to see that the spine is in alignment with the towel. Make adjustments to the towel as needed.

When your moist heat pack is in the correct position, you can assist your Receiver in laying back down on the moist heat pack.

The temperature you normally use for a moist heat pack when a Receiver is lying face down may be too hot for someone lying on it. It may be good to use two layers of dry towel between your Receiver's back and the moist hot towel. You could also just allow that moist hot towel to cool before making the moist heat pack sandwich.

(Picture #28)

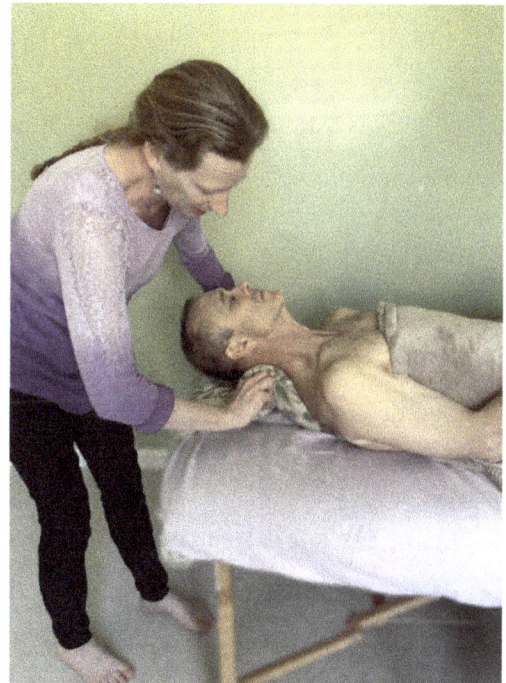

I recommend rolling up the towels by the head to make a 'moist heat pack' pillow that will sit in your Receiver's neck curve. This will also allow their neck to have moist heat on it, and it feels so good! (Picture #28)

Roll Over:

(Picture #29)

The second option is to ask your Receiver to roll over and lay on their side so that you can lay out the moist heat pack for them. So you can see their spine, you will then need to pull back the sheet to expose their back, from neck to waist. The next step is to make a 'moist heat pack sandwich' on the table and then have them lay back on it. To make this easy, lay the dry towel down parallel to your Receiver's back. Half of the dry towel should be on the table, while the other half should be hanging off the side. (Picture #29)

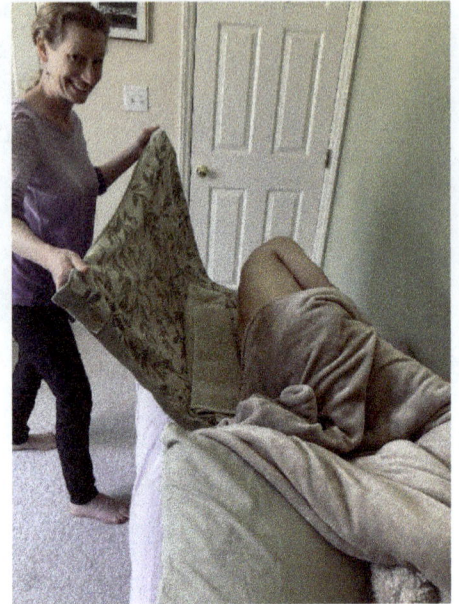

Next, lay out the hot moist towel and then use the remaining half of the dry towel to cover the moist towel.

Keep in mind that the moist heat pack will probably feel warmer to your Receiver since now their body weight is on the hot pack. You might consider laying your towels so that there are two dry towel layers on top of the moist towel.

When it is time for the Receiver to lay on the moist heat pack, I go one step further to ensure that my Receiver's spine is actually on the moist towel. I place one hand on the towel where the small of their back will lay and the other hand where their neck will be. When they lay on their back again, the moist heat pack and my hands will be under their spine. Having my hands under them momentarily will keep that heat pack from sliding around, and I'll also be able to feel with the top of my hands if the pack is under their spine. This also gives me another indication of how hot those towels are. Due to the curvature of the low back and neck, it is super easy for me to pull my hands out.

If this one step with your hands under your Receiver's body feels awkward, weird and uncomfortable, don't feel like you have to do this! It is just an extra suggestion.

Just like a moist heat pack pillow, roll up the extra towel to create a neck pillow that will offer moist heat to the cervical region of your Receiver's spine.

From here, your job is done. Your Receiver can lay on that moist heat pack without their sinuses being stuffy and painful!

Rolling over like this is a good option for those who may have difficulty sitting up.

Raindropper Tips:

If your Receiver is comfortable lying face down for an additional ten minutes, then apply that moist heat pack without concerns. If your Receiver does seem a bit stuffy, you might consider using one of these tips from fellow Raindroppers who shared what they do when their Receiver has stuffy sinuses.

Leslie Vornholt: A drop of peppermint or eucalyptus on a cotton pad that they can breathe in while face down on the table.

Carolyn McCrary: When laying on their stomach with the moist heat pack, I'll VitaFlex the sinus reflexes at the neck of toes. When they get up, I'll VitaFlex the sinuses on the forehead and sinus areas across the cheeks. Usually opens them immediately.

Lisa Storm: Our instructor said to put an oil such as RC®/Raven® blend behind the ear. Massage neck with eucalyptus so they can smell it.

Notes Page:

To watch this video on these adaptations, just request a link to the videos here:
https://adaptingraindrop.com/oilyfamvideos/

When a Receiver's Sinuses are Stuffy from Lying Face Down

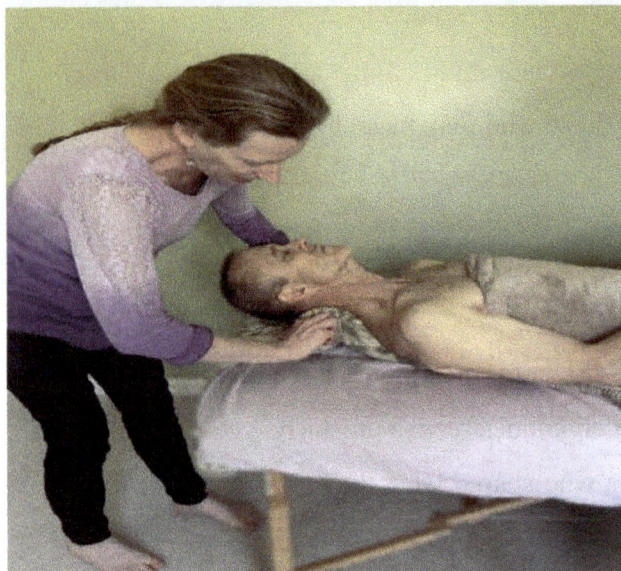

Side-lying application of moist heat pack

- Use one hand at sacrum and one hand at neck to make sure towel is along spine.
- Double up towel under neck.

Face up application of moist heat pack

- Females can use arms to hold sheets/blankets.
- Assist in sitting up and down.
- Double up towel under neck.

Tips

- Consider strength of Receiver for choosing side-lying or sitting up.
- Ask Receiver to move down before they flip over.

Notes:

_____

_____

_____

_____

_____

_____

_____

_____

_____

Chapter Nine: Giving Raindrop During Pregnancy

Why Modify for Pregnancy

A pregnant woman can receive Raindrop, but we need to adapt a few things for a mama. The adaptations will depend on what stage of pregnancy she is in. Not only do we need to look at the oils that are used, but we also need to adapt how she lays when she receives her Raindrop.

Lying Face Up

The guidance I share is from Carol Osborne-Sheets, from her book *'Pre- and Perinatal Massage Therapy'*. She recommends that once a woman has reached twenty-two weeks of her pregnancy, she should NOT lay on their back for an extended period. Carol says 'extended' is more than five minutes!

Her reasoning for why a mama should not be lying on their back for over five minutes is because the weight of the fetus could be putting pressure on the super vena cava, which is the main vein for bringing the blood back to mama's heart. If there is compression on the vein, it will affect the mom's blood pressure and the baby's.

Carol's other reason for recommending that mama does not lay on her back at this stage of pregnancy is because it can cause low back pain.

So this means that we need to adapt how we offer this mama foot VitaFlex!

Lying Face Down

Carol also recommends that once mamas reach thirteen weeks, they should NOT lay prone or on their stomachs for a long time, more than five minutes.

In '*Pre- and Perinatal Massage Therapy*', Carol explains that even though mamas may lay on their stomachs when sleeping, they should not lay on their stomachs on a massage table.

Her first reason is that when you compare the firmness of a bed versus a typical massage table, there is a big difference in how hard they are and how much they 'give'. Massage tables, even with padding, are going to be more firm with less give than a bed.

Her second reason is that when you are lying on a bed sleeping, no one puts pressure on your back. Even with Raindrop, we do put some pressure on mama's back.

This means that we will need to adapt the second half of Raindrop for mamas. This is when Receivers lie face down, and the techniques are done on the back.

When I'm working with a pregnant woman, I always err on the side of 'safer'. I choose to adapt mama's positioning on the massage table for the whole Raindrop experience. After twenty weeks of pregnancy, she will not be laying on her back for foot VitaFlex or after thirteen weeks of pregnancy laying on her stomach for the second half of Raindrop.

This is how we will do it and keep mama comfortable and safe for the whole Raindrop experience!

Adaptations for Pregnancy

Foot VitaFlex:

The easiest way to give a good Foot VitaFlex for a pregnant mom is to do this part sitting. I explain how to do this in Chapter 7.

Once you are done with Foot VitaFlex, then mama can get cozy comfortable on the massage table for the second half of her Raindrop experience. To do that, mama will go side-lying.

Side-Lying:

You can see in picture #30 that when someone is lying on their side, this is not a comfortable position to be laying in at all!

So instead, we'll use some pillows to get mama comfortable.

I bet the mama you are giving this Raindrop to may already know how to lay side-lying. This position is recommended to mamas by doctors and midwives. As her belly grows, this is the only way a mama will be able to get comfortable when sleeping! She most likely has all the pillows necessary for getting prompted up and positioned on the massage table because she uses them for sleeping. If she doesn't already know how to use these pillows to get comfortable, she will be so appreciative to learn how to get comfortable and have a good night's sleep!

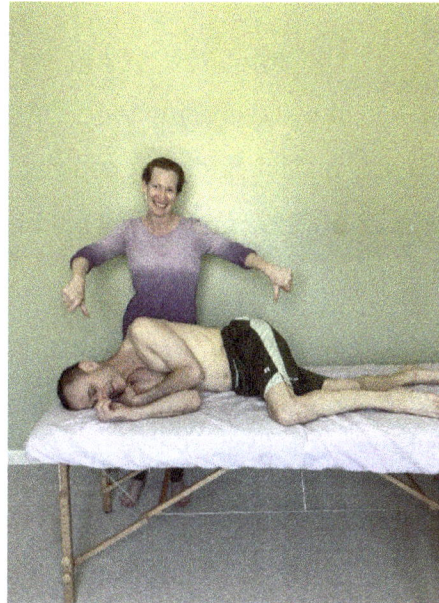

You'll need three to four pillows.

Pregnancy and Raindrop:

It is recommended that mama lay on her left side. Laying on the left allows for the best cardiac functioning of the mom, which will give the baby the most oxygen.

When mama is lying on her side, you'll place the first pillow under her head. This will keep her neck in alignment with her spine. The goal is to get mama's full spine, back and neck parallel with the massage table. The second pillow will go between her knees to keep her legs parallel. Keeping that top leg parallel with the bottom leg, instead of leaning downward, will help to avoid low back pain.

The last pillow will go by mama's chest, which she can hug on to. Hugging onto the pillow does two things. One, it helps keep mama's shoulder in good posture, so it is not falling forward. Two, it offers her additional modesty by covering her breasts.

You can see in picture #31 how those pillows allow your Receiver to lay on their side comfortably. Not only will mama be comfortable, in good alignment, in a position protecting mama and baby, but you also have access to her back!

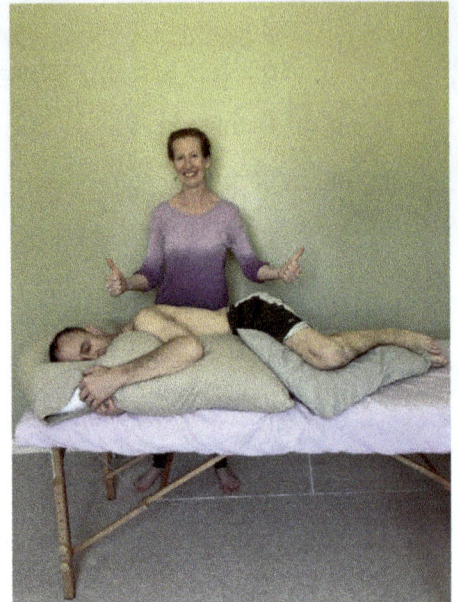

Depending on how big mama's belly is, you may also consider placing a small pillow, wedge or rolled-up blanket or towel under mama's belly. This will stop her heavy belly from hanging sideways for a long time. That can get uncomfortable too.

(Picture #32)

Don't forget, mama most likely has been using a pillow like this to help her get comfortable for sleeping. She probably knows what to do with all these pillows, but if not, you can give her some coaching and then allow her to get cozy on the massage table. Of course, you'll keep her covered with the sheet. The only part that will be exposed is her back, where you'll be dropping the oils and featuring them. In picture #32, you can see Brian's back is exposed, and I can get to it easily. I put the extra sheet on his shoulder and tucked the sheet into his pants so it would not move.

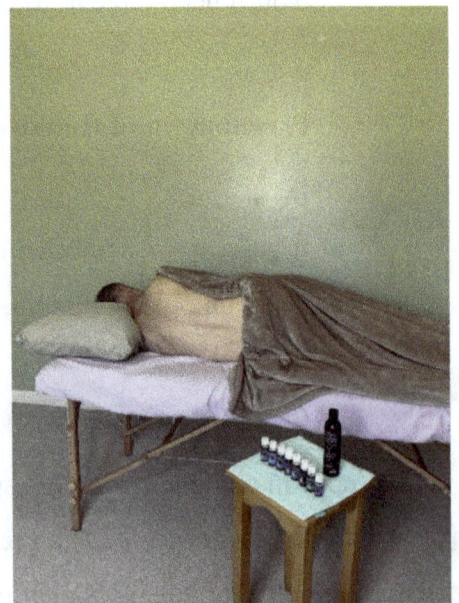

You may have seen the nifty pregnancy pillows just for massaging women when they are pregnant. The pillows have cutouts for swollen breasts and bellies. The idea is with these cutouts in the pillow; mama can lay face down comfortably on a massage table without her belly getting in the way. I'm not a fan of these pregnancy pillows, and neither is Carol. She explains that when a pregnant mama lays face down on one of these pillows, it causes further strain on the taxed uterine ligaments.

Another consideration is these pregnancy pillows with cutouts are super expensive. There is no need for this extra expense. You can set up mama to be toasty and comfortable with the adaptations I will share with you here.

(Picture #33)

Dropping Oils and Doing Techniques:

When you drop oils along a back that is side-lying, it will be very different compared to dropping oils on a back that is lying prone. In side-lying, gravity is working against us. You'll notice that when you drop an oil, the drop quickly rolls down towards the massage table. You'll need to be flexible in this situation and drop above the spine, knowing that they will cross the spine and head towards the table. (Picture #33)

It is best to work quickly, drop those oils and start feathering right away!

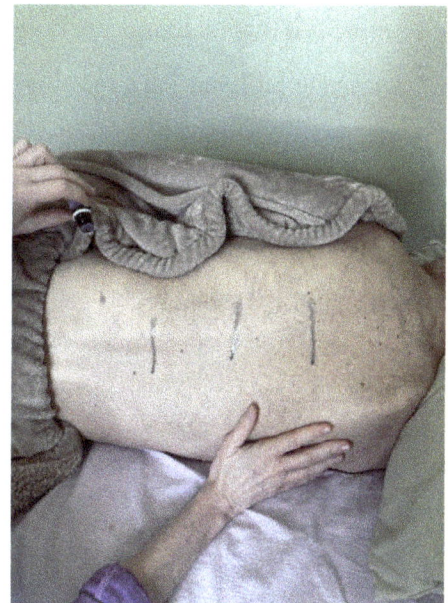

You can do all the techniques that are normally done in Raindrop. You just need to modify or adapt the technique and your body posture to get it all done.

Finger Circles

You will need to be on your knees to get to the correct angle. You'll simply walk on your knees to move from sacrum to skull.

As always, when doing this technique, you are not going to push muscles against or towards the spine. You will only push muscle away from the spine.   (Picture #34)

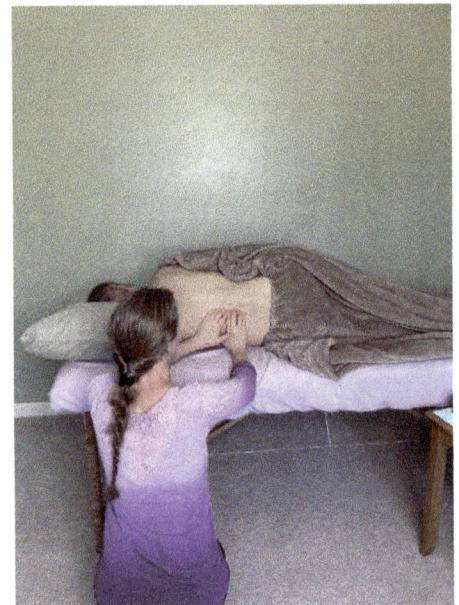

When making the finger circles, you will need to approach this technique as if you are standing on one side of the massage table and not moving from the right to the left side, as commonly taught in Raindrop classes. In this case, on the side of the spine closest to the massage table, your finger circles will have a 'pull' as you rotate your fingers towards the table. (Picture #34)

(Picture #35)

To do finger circles on the other side of the spine, the side that is furthest away from the massage table, will be the circle toward the ceiling with the 'pull' to it. (Picture #35)

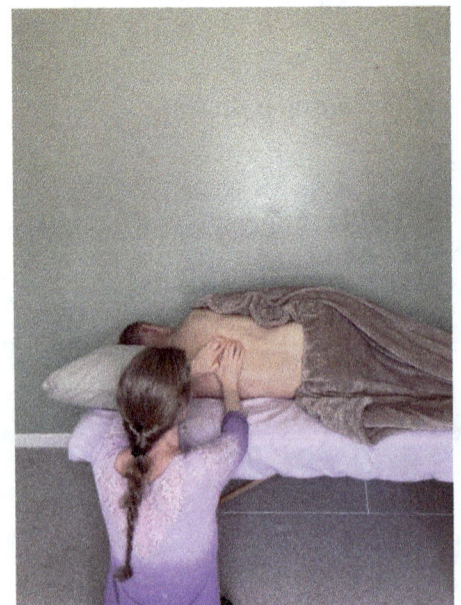

(Picture #36)

Thumb VitaFlex

This technique will be done the same way with your thumbs. The only difference is your posture. The adaptation for this technique is you will need to have a wide base which will allow you to work lower. You create a wide base by having a wide stance, as in picture #36. You will simply take steps in this wide stance to move from sacrum to skull.

You don't want to bend over to work lower on the massage table. If you find yourself bending over the massage table a lot when doing Raindrop, I suggest you get 'Pain-Free Raindrop'. This online program will teach you how to stand and move at a massage table without YOUR neck or back hurting.

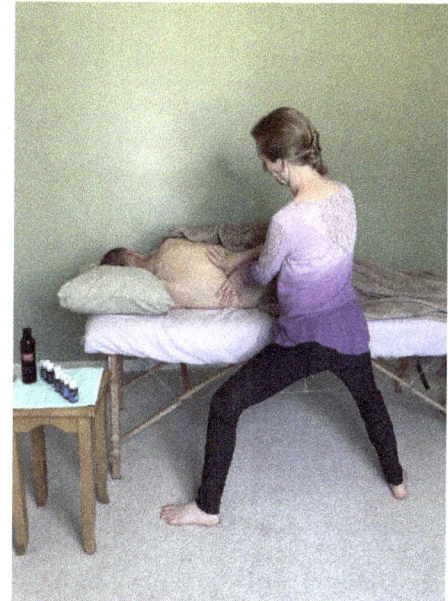

(Picture #37)

Saw Maneuver

Saw Maneuver will be done the same way; it is just your stance that will be different. It is best to do this technique on your knees. (Picture #37). You'll notice that there will not be as much rocking back and forth as to when this technique is done face down. Do your best to follow the natural rhythm of your Receiver instead of forcing your rocking rhythm on them.

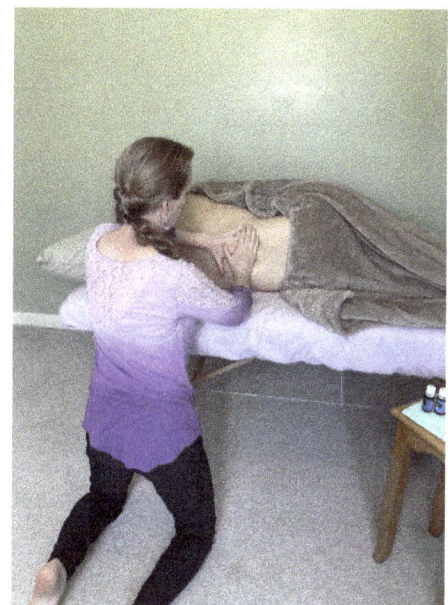

Stretch and Rock

Again, this technique will be done the same way, but you must change your posture. This technique will also be done on your knees. You will notice, like, in Saw Maneuver, your Receiver will not shake or rock as much.

(Picture #38)

Palm Slide

This is a technique that will be abbreviated because we can't reach the full-back. You can still get tissue movement and should try to. The lower you are to do this technique, the stronger you will be; the kneeling position is best for you to do this. (Picture #38)

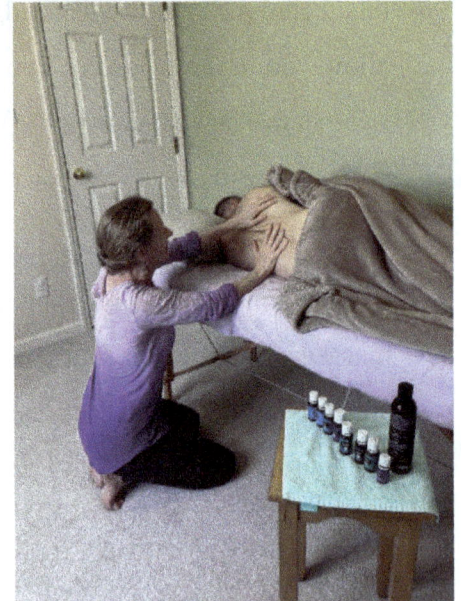

(Picture #39)

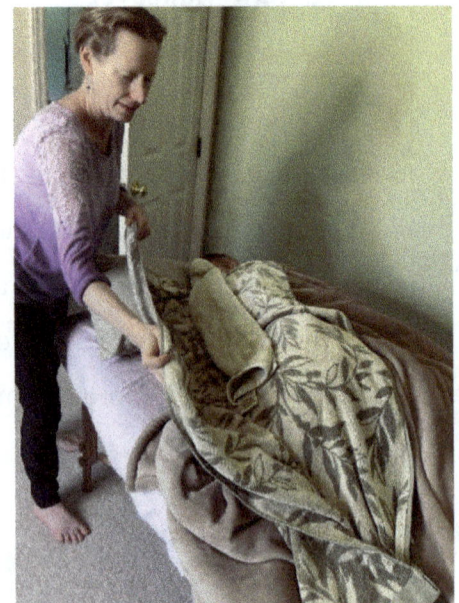

Moist Heat Pack

Applying the moist heat pack will be similar to when your Receiver is lying on their stomach. The only difference is you are putting the towels on a sideways surface, and they may slide down a bit. To stop the towels from sliding, you can put a corner of the first layer of dry towel over your Receiver's shoulder and hip. (Picture #39)

The rest of the moist heat pack sandwich is the same. Roll out the hot moist towel along the spine. The weight of the second dry towel stops the moist towel from sliding. Then cover with the sheet and if you want, add an additional blanket for extra warmth. (Picture #40).

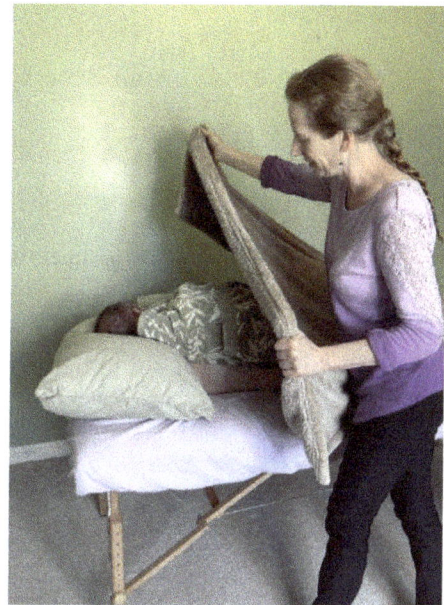

(Picture #41)

Removing the moist heat pack will be done the same way as if your Receiver was laying on their stomach. Simply hold the blanket and sheet while the other hand pulls out the moist heat pack. This allows mama to stay covered with sheet and blanket during and after removing the moist heat pack sandwich. (Picture #41)

As we were taking these videos, my husband, who was my demo, was so comfortable in this side-lying position that he fell asleep! There is no reason that you should worry that your side-lying Receiver will be uncomfortable.

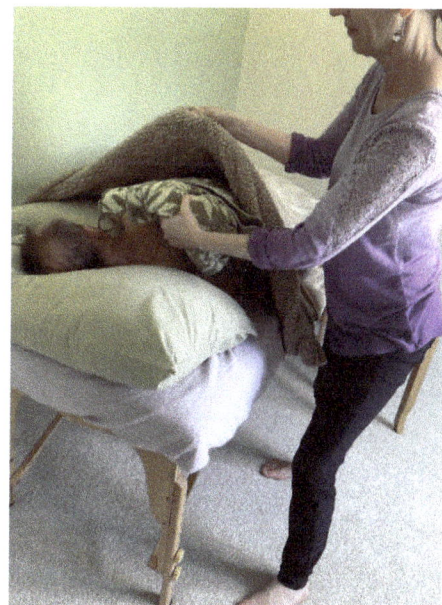

Getting Up

At some point, your Receiver will have to get up off that cozy, warm massage table. I have some tips for you to make it easier for her to get up and allow you to be with her the whole time.

The first thing to do is remove the pillow between her knees and remove the pillow she was hugging on to. Since mama is covered with a sheet or blanket, you'll want to remove these pillows while keeping her covered and warm. (Picture #42)

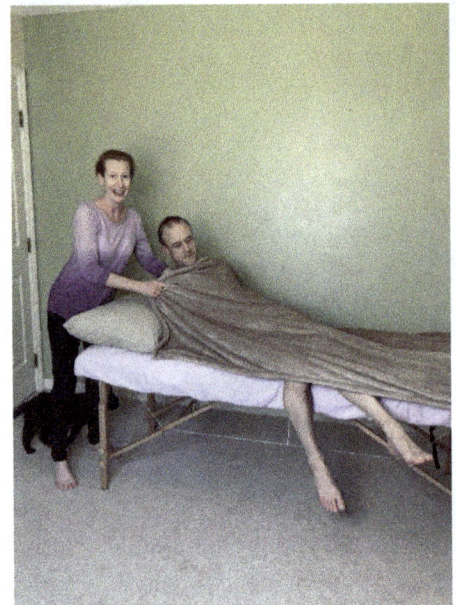

Then instruct her to swing her legs to the side of the massage table. While she is doing that, you will hold the sheet up by her shoulder, so it stays there to keep her front covered. (Picture #42)

(Picture #43)

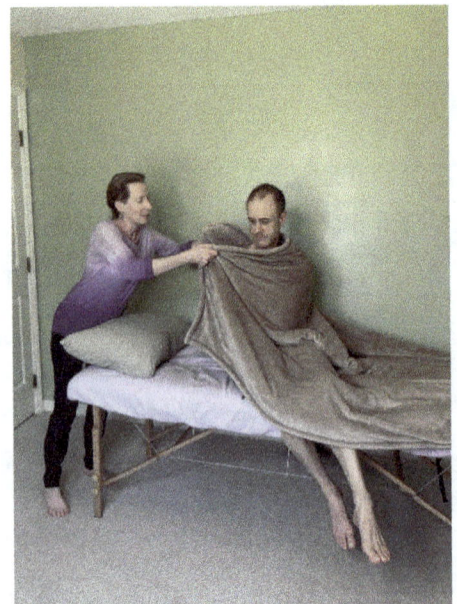

Keep on holding that sheet to her shoulder. As she is getting up, you can reach behind her with your other hand, grab the sheet by her other shoulder and bring the two ends of the sheet together. (Picture #43)

She is now fully wrapped up by the sheet. This keeps her warm and modest.

Now, with mama fully covered and sitting on the table, you can check in with her and see how she is doing. (Picture #44)

When ready, she can hop off the massage table, get dressed and have a glass of water.

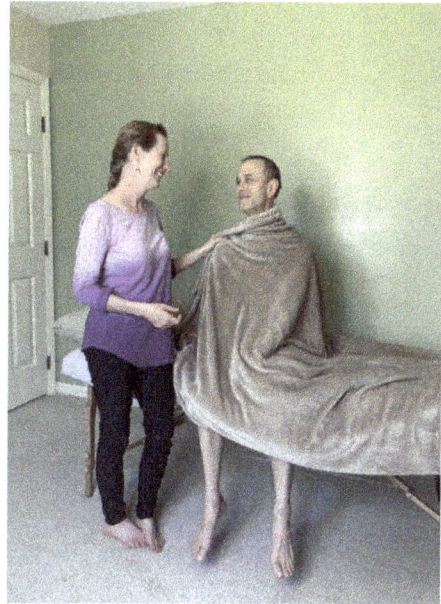

Notes Page:

To watch this video on these adaptations, just request a link to the videos here:

https://adaptingraindrop.com/oilyfamvideos/

Giving Raindrops during Pregnancy

Tips

- At 13 weeks or more, mama should not lay on back or stomach for Raindrop. Instead use side-lying position.
- Use pillow to align head and neck with spine.
- Use pillow between knees to keep legs parallel so lower back does not hurt.
- Use pillow for mama to 'hug on to' for comfort and to lean forward a bit.
- For all techniques, Giver uses a low, wide stance or works on knees.
- Apply moist heat pack in traditional manner.
- Help mama up and use sheet to keep her covered.

Foot VitaFlex

- Do this sitting.
- Keep Receiver's foot lower to keep Giver in good posture.

Notes:

_____

_____

_____

_____

_____

_____

_____

_____

_____

Chapter Ten: Giving Raindrop To Babies And Toddlers

Yes, you can give a Raindrop to babies and toddlers! I gave my daughter many Raindrops when she was just a little baby. I learned quite a lot as I gave her these Raindrops. I continued to use those adaptive techniques into her toddler years too.

You will need to adapt the Raindrop experience for your little ones. It is a good idea to think about your oil choices and dilution when working with little guys. To get dilution ratios and oil ideas, go to 'Special Considerations' in this book. That will discuss more of those topics. Another good resource is *'Gentle Babies'* by Debra Reyburn.

This chapter is all about practical tips on how to give a Raindrop to babies and toddlers.

You will need to change things up for giving Raindrop because a little one, especially a toddler, will not lay still for a full hour while you give them a Raindrop like an adult. I don't think there is any reason why we should expect little guys to lay on a massage table, bed, or floor for an extended period while we apply oils on their backs. I have some great tips to share that will make this Raindrop with babies and toddlers a relaxing and enjoyable experience for all involved.

The Adaptations:

How do you give a Raindrop to a little squirmy baby or toddler without dropping oil bottles, babies crawling away, and toddlers crying? This is how.

The first step is to GET ORGANIZED. You should have everything that you need for this Raindrop within arm's reach. Ideally, at the end of this Raindrop, you and your little one will have time to relax, cuddle and maybe even nap together.

You will need within arm's reach:

- Base oil

- A small bowl for each oil that you will use. You will dilute your oils ahead of time and have them ready to use in the bowls.

- Warm blanket

The best time to give your little ones a Raindrop is when they are sleepy and relaxed. I have found that bath time is a perfect prelude to Raindrop. Not only does this help your little one relax and get warm, but they are also naked, and you have easy access to their back.

Get everything ready before bath time, and then when the bath is done, head to your Raindrop location. This may be a comfortable rocking chair or your bed.

(Picture #45)

Position baby over your shoulder, like if you were going to burp them. With your Raindrop tools by your side ready to use, you can reach for the base oil and apply some on your little one's back. This application of base oil will slow the absorption of the essential oil and make sure there is no discomfort from the phenols doing their job. To apply base oil, just put a few drops in one hand and rub it on the baby's back. (Picture #45)

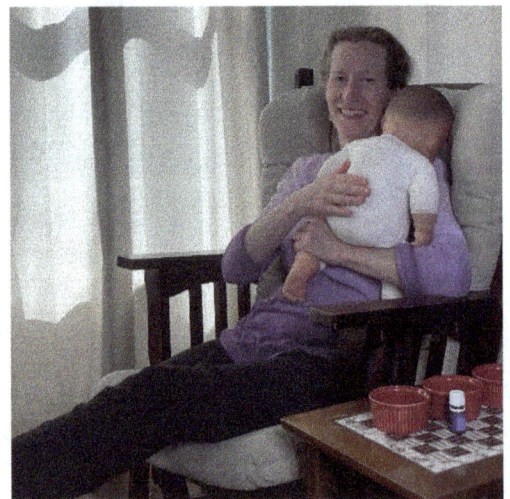

82

The Essential Oil Application:

You have your essential oil and base oil blended in the small bowls to the dilution you decide on. Each essential oil you choose will be mixed with a base oil in an individual bowl. You just need to dip the fingers of one hand in a bowl and then apply that blend on baby's back by feathering it in. (Picture #46)

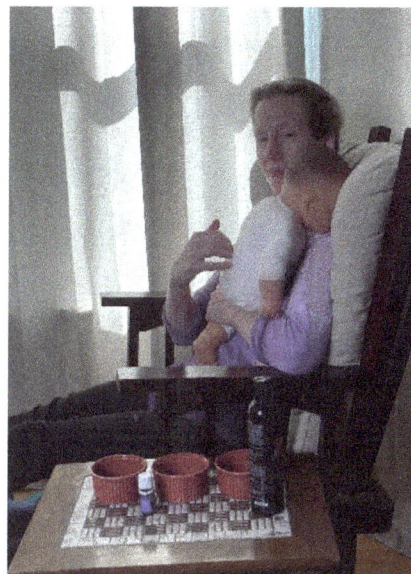

That feathering will be calming for the baby, just like it is for you. You may not be using your nails to feather as we teach for adults, but your feathering will stimulate the baby's nerves exiting her spine. The baby is getting all the benefits of Raindrop; essential oils and nerve stimulation. The slower your feathering is, the more calming and relaxing it is for the baby!

Do that with each oil you choose to use.

Picture #47

If you want and your little one is up for more, you can also do some gentle finger circles. In picture #47, I am doing finger circles on the baby's left side. I can easily do finger circles on the baby's right side by moving my hand/fingers to the other side of her spine. Remember, the 'pull' will always be away from the spine.

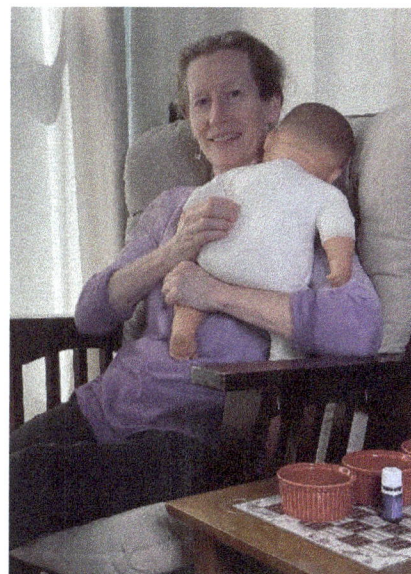

This is more relaxing the slower your circles are. You can do each side one time, two times, or three times. See how receptive your little one is.

Other techniques typically used in Raindrop will not be used here. You can always do some large circles with your palm on the baby's back. Who doesn't find that super relaxing?

I'm going to suggest you skip the moist heat pack too. Instead, grab that warm blanket and cover up yourself and your baby. (Picture #48) Now, the two of you can just take a nap together.

In the pictures, I was sitting in a rocking chair. You can also do this laying on a bed with your little one on your tummy. Another option is if you are both laying on your sides, like when nursing. In the cold winter, I sat on the toilet in the bathroom because I didn't want to leave the warm bathroom. Once the Raindrop was done, it was easy to move to the bed and cover up with more blankets. As with anything when it comes to little ones, be flexible and do what works for the two of you!

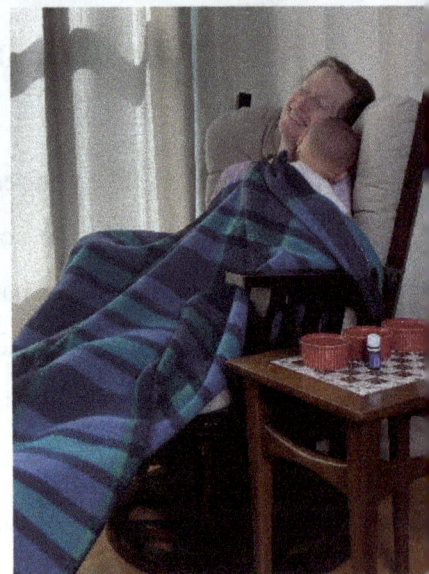

Toddlers:

You can still use this same method as your baby grows into a toddler. You may not be holding your toddler up on your shoulder, but they can sit facing you on your lap with their legs on either side. This will give you access to their back for the Raindrop and some wonderful cuddling time.

Notes Page:

To watch this video on these adaptations, just request a link to the videos here:

https://adaptingraindrop.com/oilyfamvideos/

Giving Raindrops to Babies and Toddlers

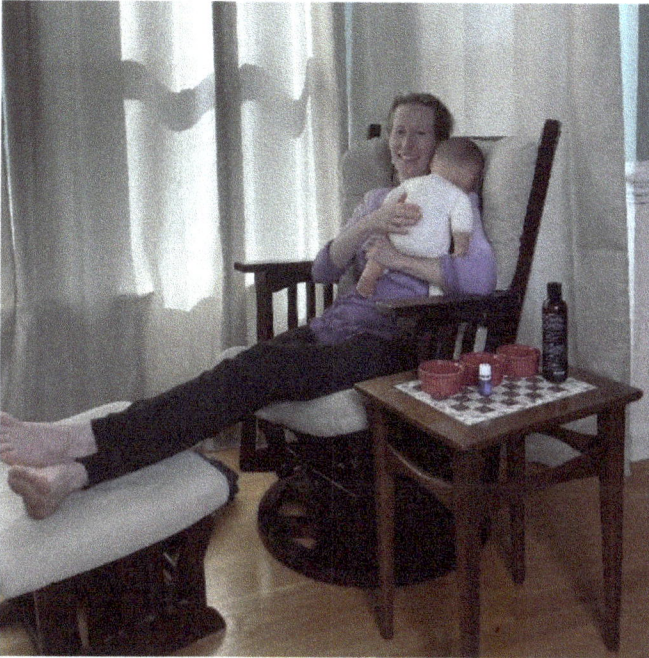

Tips

- Get everything ready ahead of time.
  - Base oil
  - Diluted oil
  - Blanket
- Use slower techniques, they are more relaxing for baby.
- Instead of moist heat pack, cover up baby and yourself with blanket and take some time to rest.
- Toddlers can sit on your lap facing you.

Notes:

_____

_____

_____

_____

_____

_____

_____

_____

_____

Part 3

Special Considerations

Chapter Eleven: Special Considerations

This is not a fully inclusive list, and it is not meant to be. I didn't intend this chapter to be like the *Essential Oils Desk Reference* because chapter 1-5 gives you the tools to tailor your Raindrops for many common wellness concerns.

This chapter is meant to share tips, adaptations, or stories to help you add or modify your Raindrops when giving them to someone with a 'special consideration'.

These tips have come from light-bulb moments as I worked with clients and family. Some of these tips are stories that I thought you'd be interested in because they taught me a huge lesson! Some of these tips have come from other Raindroppers, and I'm passing them on.

This is a chapter that I envision will be growing as more people read this resource guide. I'd love for you to send me your tips and stories on how you adapted a Raindrop to support a unique need. You can always submit a tip or story here: AdaptingRaindrop.com

As I receive your tips and stories, I'll add them in the new edition, and with your permission, I would like to give you credit.

I put these tips in alphabetical order to make them easier to find.

Many of these 'special considerations' can be hot topics. I have seen them create discourse and disagreement because there are so many views regarding essential oil use. My tips and feelings on these special considerations are not the only views but take and use what feels good and right to you.

Amputation

I have not had the opportunity to use this tip yet, but it makes so much sense when you learn about our body's energy field. The tip is when working with someone who is experiencing phantom pain after an amputation, do VitaFlex as if the limb was there. It has been reported that VitaFlexing the aura of the missing limb eliminated phantom pain for some Receivers. When combining oils and Vita Flex, there is so much energy involved in Raindrop; it does not surprise me that these techniques would help restore the connection of a wounded aura.

Autism

The Autism Spectrum is wide, and once again, each person who has been diagnosed is unique.

As with each Receiver, it is imperative that you apply the information gained in Part 1. Ask those questions and consider the concepts to determine how much oil and perhaps which oils to use. It may be more appropriate to ask the mother or caregiver these questions and explain the concepts behind each question.

My experience giving Raindrop to kids on the spectrum has always been pleasantly positive. During our time together, moms were always surprised at how well their child enjoyed Raindrop.

A common behavior of those diagnosed with severe autism is tactile sensitivity, sensitivity to new types of touch or textures, and not wanting to be touched, especially by a new person. Another common behavior of those on the spectrum is desiring constant movement.

Both of these common behaviors, tactile sensitivity and need for movement, seem to negate that whole idea of giving someone a Raindrop who has severe autism. I have given this technique to three young clients diagnosed with severe autism, who received it willingly with enjoyment.

What I did was skip the foot Vita Flex and start with feathering on the back. I decided to skip working on the feet because feet tend to be an extremely sensitive area. Lying face down always helps my adult clients relax, so I thought this would help these boys too; it did.

Before we started, I told the boys that they were in total control of how long they stayed on the massage table. I let them know that when they wanted Raindrop to stop, all they needed to say was "I'm all done", and they were free to get up. This worked well, and they stayed on the table longer than I expected.

The feathering technique is magic and does a wonderful job at stimulating the parasympathetic nervous system, which supports the body's systems to relax. All three of these kids loved the feathering techniques and voluntarily stayed still on the table for twenty to forty-five minutes. This time of peaceful relaxation was appreciated by both their moms and the boys. As they became more comfortable with Raindrop with repeat visits, their time on the table increased.

Babies

Babies are small, and their systems are new and more sensitive than a child or adults. The big key to remember for babies is to dilute, decrease and go slow.

Start with diluting at least 50/50.
Use one to two oils and see how the baby responds.

Are you going to do a full Raindrop on a baby? No way, but you can use this technique to apply oils to these little bodies and see wonderful results.

Most babies would receive Raindrop to support their digestive system, respiratory system, immune system, or to help them relax.

Keep in mind that when you are massaging your baby, the slower the movements are, the more relaxing they are. This is a wonderful way to cuddle with the baby and take some time for both of you to relax and nap.

For detailed information, go to Chapter 10, 'Giving Raindrop to Babies and Toddlers'.

Brain

For those Receivers who need support for their brain function, such as with Traumatic Brain Injury (TBI), Down syndrome, stroke, or Parkinson's Disease, I'd like to share a tip that I received from Dr. David Stewart. He suggested that when you are doing feathering, instead of stopping at the occipitals or base of the skull, keep on feathering the head up to the Receiver's crown or top of the head.

Do this extended feathering for each oil and each time you do feathering.

Consider using oils that support oxygenation and oils that target that Receiver's specific needs/goals.

Cancer

This is a topic that has many opinions and views. Thank you for letting me express mine here.

If someone has been diagnosed with cancer, it is very important that you discuss the detoxing questions with them in chapter 2 and modify your Raindrop accordingly.

Anyone who has received this diagnosis is most certainly full of emotions. This path contains countless questions and decisions that develop into a unique journey. Not everyone is going to make the choices you would make.

It is paramount that as a Raindropper, you need to educate your Receiver and allow them to be involved in the decisions and goals regarding Raindrop. It is also best for you to work with the support of a Natural Wellness Professional who is open to essential oils and Raindrop. The Receiver should be a patient of this Wellness Professional, and they can guide you in oil choices and help if there is a detox reaction. Raindrop itself is not a cure-all, but it can greatly support our wellness goals.

> **"The client has the final say. Education is a must."**
>
> Kristi Zittle

I've worked with clients that once they received the cancer diagnosis, they started a dramatic cleansing and detox protocol with medical support. They were doing daily colon cleanses and eating clean, and their body was prepared to manage additional toxins the phenols kicked up during their Raindrop. They were ready for additional cleansing and came to me with that intention.

I've also worked with clients diagnosed with cancer who were very sickly, and their body was not ready to process any toxic load. With this client, I saw my primary role was to support their lymphatic system so it could allow the body to remove the toxic overload their body was holding onto.

In the Adapting Raindrop Facebook group, Sherian McCoy shared a helpful tip that I was unaware of. She said, "I am a holistic cancer coach and do Raindrop frequently on patients undergoing chemo. The rule of thumb is to keep the Raindrop for forty-eight hours on either side of the chemo days. It is not recommended for those undergoing radiation."

A bit of advice that I have carried with me and applied often is from Marie Koepke, RN. She explained to me that someone who has cancer is someone whose body is not dealing with detox well. When looking at it this way, it does not make sense to ask a body already having difficulty processing toxins to add essential oils, which will 'kick up' more toxins to be processed. Their body has difficulty processing toxins; why add oils that will overwhelm the system. Instead, use oils that will support the body with healing by choosing to use oils that are high in monoterpenes and sesquiterpenes.

Children

Depending on how big your kiddo is and how cuddly they are, you can use the adaptations for giving Raindrop to babies for a long time.

For children, you will still decrease, dilute and go slow. If this is a child's first time receiving oils on their back, then applying a base oil first is highly suggested. You will not be doing a full Raindrop session on a child, which is fine. Choose two to four oils that will support your goals.

Children usually receive Raindrops for respiratory support, immune support, digestive support, and relaxation.

Some kids will lay there and enjoy all the relaxing and stimulating tactile stimulation, while others will not. Just go with it and be flexible. Don't force it. Just remember, your primary goal is to get the oils on! With children, you are definitely going to be doing a 'Quickie Raindrop'. Any other gentle rubbing, finger circles, spinal Vital Flex you get in is icing on the cake.

For more information on how to give Raindrop to children, go to Chapter 10, 'Giving Raindrop to Babies and Toddlers'.

Cortisone Injections for Pain

People typically get cortisone or steroid injections to relieve joint pain. These shots reduce inflammation in the area and calm the nerves, which often reduces the pain. What we want to remember when it comes to Raindrop in relation to these injections is that the injection needs to stay in the body for a few days to do its job. We don't want the essential oils from Raindrop to break down the steroid before it has the chance to complete its goal.

The common recommendation for going back to exercise after the injection is three to ten days.

Massage is generally not recommended right after receiving a steroid or cortisone injection. Leaning towards the conservative side, it is a good idea to wait seven to fourteen days after the injection to do a Raindrop.

Digestive System

To support your Receiver's colon and get those exits working well, you can add some extra VitaFlex along with the colon points on the shin and sole of the feet. (Both of these locations and techniques are taught in CARE VitaFlex classes).

For myself and my family, I have simply applied one to three oils along the lower spine with some feathering to work with the nerves that support the digestive system. In this way, I'm harnessing the power of the 'Nerve Pathway Subway System' to deliver those oils right where they are needed.

Tanya Schoessow also shared, "For those needing extra digestive support, after VitaFlexing the legs and feet, I'll apply a warm towel to the shins. The Receiver is given a huge WOW after ;)"

Multiple Sclerosis (MS) and Other Conditions Affect the Myelin Sheath

What happens with MS is that the myelin sheath that covers the nerve gets inflamed, which causes scars. This damage to the myelin sheath results in a poor connection or no connection between the Central Nervous System and muscles served by that nerve.

Heat makes MS symptoms worse by further reducing the ability of the nerves to conduct electrical impulses. Instead of applying a moist heat pack at the end of Raindrop, apply a cool or cold pack.

If you are not sure or feel guilty about putting a cool pack on your Receiver, ask them a simple question, "Do you prefer to take hot or cool showers?" Their response will guide you in what temperature pack to use.

Nursing

There are three questions that nursing mamas ask when it comes to nursing and Raindrop.

1. Mama usually wonders if the peppermint in Raindrop will reduce her milk production.

2. Mama wants to know if the oils will change the taste of her milk.

3. Mama is concerned that she will detox from the Raindrop, and the toxins will go into her milk.

Let's address each concern.

1. "Will peppermint reduce my milk?"

There is a 50/50 chance that peppermint will reduce a nursing mama's milk. If my Receiver is a new mama and she is anxious about the possibility of reducing her milk, then I simply omit peppermint and use another oil instead; rosemary or copaiba. My philosophy is, why cause any more stress for a new mom?

If the Receiver is an experienced mama and is open to testing out how her body responds to peppermint when nursing, I'll use it. It is important to educate mama and leave the decision entirely up to her.

2. "Will the oils change the taste of my milk?"

When used in Raindrop, I feel that essential oils will add a slight flavor to mama's milk. Any foods we eat will affect the quality, color, and taste of our milk!

When I was nursing and giving Raindrops, my girl never turned up her nose at my milk, even when giving or receiving a Raindrop. Many nursing mamas have reported that their baby did not slow down nursing after mama had their Raindrop. Actually, once my girl started eating solid foods, she enjoyed a wide variety of flavors and spices. I wonder if my essential oil use contributed to her being open to a wide range of flavors.

If there is still a concern, then mama should be encouraged to do a small test. She can apply some of the more flavorful oils like oregano, thyme, and basil to her feet and see how the baby responds when nursing a few hours later. Perhaps she just experiences Foot VitaFlex with all the Raindrop oils and then observes the baby's nursing behavior for the next day or two. After these tests, mama can then make an informed and confident decision about receiving a full Raindrop.

3. "If I detox from Raindrop, will the toxins go into my milk?"

Sadly, since we have been exposed to so many toxins throughout the years, toxins have been found in breast milk. But, having a Raindrop does not mean your body will be disposing of the toxins your body releases into your breast milk.

Since the mammary glands and lymph nodes are so close to each other in the breast tissue and axillary region (underarm), people seem to worry that they are similar systems or will easily 'mix', which is not the case at all! Your body eliminates toxins through the lymphatic system, and a nursing mama produces milk in mammary glands.

Mammary glands are enlarged and modified sweat glands. Mammary glands are hollow cavities (alveoli) lined with milk-secreting cells. Mammary glands are regulated by mama's hormones, the endocrine system, NOT the lymphatic system.

The lymphatic system is an open system. It is made of liquid that bathes all our cells. The lymph's job is to collect large molecules like toxins, dead cells, and bacteria and carry these into the lymph vessels. Lymph vessels travel from fingers and toes to the heart. Along the lymph vessels are lymph nodes, where white blood cells wait to attack and destroy what was brought into the lymph vessels.

Lymph nodes are part of the lymphatic system; they are NOT part of the endocrine system.

Even though lymph nodes and mammary glands both look like little hollow balls and are found in the breast, they are not regulated by the same system. If mama detoxed from Raindrop, there is no reason for mama's body to eliminate toxins through her breast milk; her lymph system would do that job.

Should mama go on a big detox while nursing? I don't think that is a wise idea because her body needs more calories and nutrition to produce enough milk. Paying attention to the quality and purity of her food while pregnant and nursing is the best choice.

Staying hydrated by drinking lots of water is the best way to support mama's lymphatic system.

Asking the right questions and making adjustments if needed are still appropriate for a nursing mama.

Pregnancy

In time, that 'baby bump' makes it uncomfortable and even unsafe for mama to lay on her stomach. *Detailed information on how to help Mama get comfortable on a massage table in Chapter 9, 'Giving Raindrop During Pregnancy'.*

There are many views if one should receive a Raindrop when pregnant. I determined my answer based on how much essential oil the expecting mom used <u>before</u> becoming pregnant. If she did not use oils before pregnancy, my thought is, why introduce a bunch of oils at one time (as in Raindrop) now. Why not see if there are one or two oils she can use to help her find the support she is looking for. Most expectant moms are looking for support with their digestive system, muscular system, immune system, or sleep. This is where the book *Gentle Babies by Debra Rayburn* will help you find out what oils or supplements could be helpful and appropriate.

When I was pregnant, I gave Raindrops and taught CARE classes through all nine months. Now, that was a lot of essential oil I was exposing myself and my energetic baby to, but I felt comfortable doing so. I had been exposed to that amount of oil for years before pregnancy. My body was used to the oils. In fact, the only time during my nine months of pregnancy that I did not have 'morning sickness' was when I was giving a Raindrop!!

In my practice, I have a personal rule that if a mama is new to Raindrop, then I will not do a Raindrop on her in the first trimester. This is a delicate time, and if anything were to happen, I would not want her to have any thoughts at all that Raindrop or oils could have been the cause.

You may consider using a 'System Supporting Raindrop' if needed or using singles or blends that would support and prepare a mama for giving birth.

I feel strongly that when in doubt if oil should or should not be used, the mama has the final say.

Scoliosis

A common question I receive is, "If someone has scoliosis, should I do the techniques to follow their spine, or should I do the techniques in the middle of their back where the spine should be?"

Follow their spine. It is the best way to stimulate the nerves exiting the spine.

Chapter Twelve: Continue Growing

I hope you found this resource guide helpful! As I shared before, this guide is meant to grow.

My Vision Is For This Resource Guide to Grow

I'd appreciate it if you shared with me what you found worked well for you.

Do you give Raindrops to someone who has a special consideration? What have you found that works exceptionally well with them? Please share tips that you have used often with success. What do you do differently that you feel will be helpful for others in a similar situation? Let me know so that we can share it with others.

My vision is to have a library or repository of Raindrop expertise and experiences. That way, when you have a question on how to do a Raindrop on someone who is or who has, you have a resource to go for ideas.

I have started that library in two ways; one is in this book you are holding, and the second is in 'All Things Raindrop Educational Membership'. All Things Raindrop is a video library that members can access 24/7. Currently, a video is added once a week on a different topic. You'll find interviews with wellness practitioners, moms, and grandmas all sharing an experience of giving Raindrop, their observations, what they learned from it, and advice they would give to other Raindroppers.

I'm excited for you to be part of it! If you'd like to share your story feel free to contact me on my website AdaptingRaindrop.com

Chapter Thirteen: Popular Educational Programs

Some of the most popular programs and educational memberships you can find on

www.AdaptingRaindrop.com

All Things Raindrop Educational Membership

Get 24/7 access to video interviews, tips, and education that is related to Raindrop. Listen to interviews with wellness providers, Raindrop technique specialists, moms, and grandmas who share what they have learned with their experiences of giving Raindrop. Each video is filled with healthy, spiritual, oily nuggets of wisdom.

Pain-Free Raindrop Online Program

Learn how to stand at a massage table and move your body while giving a Raindrop. When you are not in pain, you'll do a better job, you'll be able to focus on your Receiver, and you'll be able to do more Raindrops!

Check AdaptingRaindrop.com for other online programs and books all related to The Raindrop Technique.

Raindrop Tools

I've been making a collection of our Favorite Oily tools so that it is easy for you to find them when you are looking for them. For each item, I'll tell you why it was added to the list.

You'll find Social Media links on AdaptingRaindrop.com Please join me to chat about Raindrop, Oils and more!

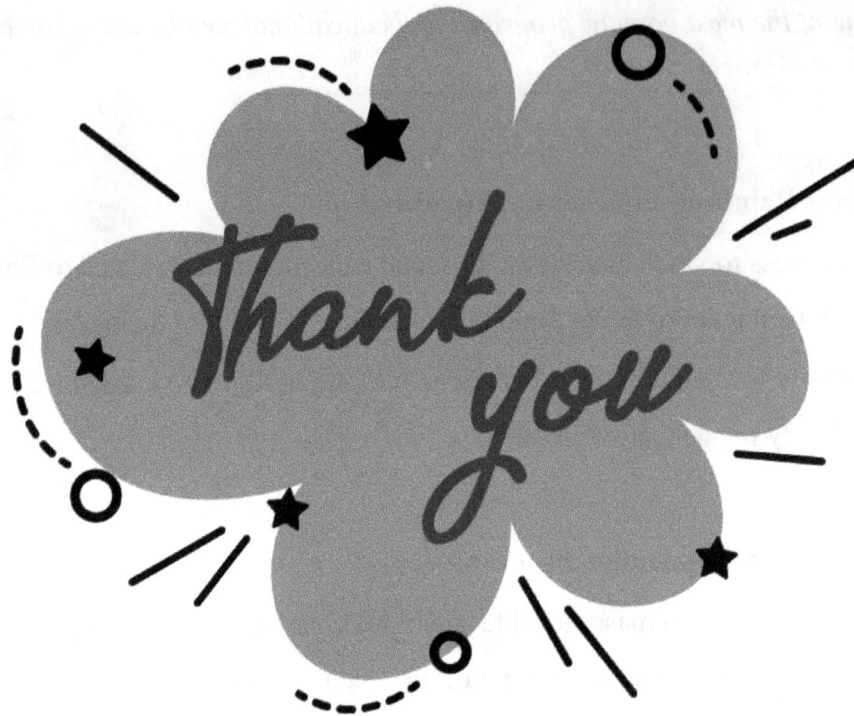

Thank You For Reading My Book!

I really appreciate all of your feedback and I love hearing what you have to say.

I need your input to make the next version of this and and my future books better.

Please take two minutes now to leave a helpful review where you purchased this book.   You also are welcome to send me an email.

Thanks so much!

Christina Hagan